Hypertension in Focus

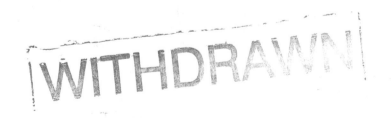

Hypertension in Focus

Susan Shankie

BPharm, MSc, MRPharmS

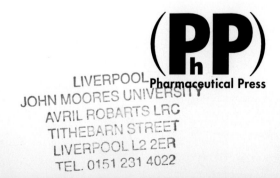

PhP Pharmaceutical Press

Published by the Pharmaceutical Press
1 Lambeth High Street, London SE1 7JN, UK

© Pharmaceutical Press 2001

First published 2001

Text design by Barker/Hilsdon, Lyme Regis, Dorset
Typeset by Type Study, Scarborough, North Yorkshire
Printed in Great Britain by TJ International, Padstow, Cornwall

ISBN 0 85369 456 7

For David and Anna

Contents

About the author

Susan Shankie graduated in 1984 from Nottingham University (BPharm) and went on to do her pre-registration year at Great Ormond Street children's hospital. She continued to work there as basic grade and staff pharmacist until August 1989 when she joined the editorial team of *Martindale: The Extra Pharmacopoeia* (published by the Pharmaceutical Press). She worked on the 30th, 31st and 32nd editions of *Martindale* until December 1998, during which time she did an MSc in Biopharmacy at King's College, London. Since 1998 Susan has worked on a freelance basis for the Pharmaceutical Press and *Martindale*.

Abbreviations

ACE	angiotensin-converting enzyme
AT1	angiotensin type 1
BHS	British Hypertension Society
CHD	coronary heart disease
ECG	electrocardiogram
HDL-cholesterol	high-density lipoprotein cholesterol
ISA	intrinsic sympathomimetic activity
JNC	Joint National Committee (US)
LDL-cholesterol	low-density lipoprotein cholesterol
MAOI	monoamine oxidase inhibitor
NSAID	non-steroidal anti-inflammatory drug
OTC	over-the-counter
SPC	summary of product characteristics
VLDL-cholesterol	very-low-density lipoprotein cholesterol
WHO/ISH	World Health Organization/International Society of Hypertension

1

Introduction

Hypertension is a massive health problem; the 1996 Health Survey for England found that about half of the people aged between 65 and 74 years had hypertension and among older people the prevalence was even higher.[1] Hypertension is one of the major risk factors for cardiovascular mortality, which is a major cause of death in the UK. It is also a major risk factor for cardiovascular morbidity that has considerable health care costs. Although cardiovascular mortality rates had been declining in some westernised countries, there is some recent evidence that this decline has decreased and, even where age-adjusted rates continue to fall, the ageing population of most developed countries means that the total numbers of cardiovascular events are typically increasing. The successful management of hypertension, both in the individual patient and at a population level, is therefore vital if the burden of cardiovascular disease is to be reduced.

Despite the availability of a wide range of drugs that are effective at lowering blood pressure, surveys[2-4] continue to reveal that those people treated for hypertension are often not controlled satisfactorily and that many people discontinue their treatment. One survey in the UK indicated that only 6% of hypertensive patients had their blood pressure lowered to <140/90 mmHg.[4] The surveys also reveal substantial underdiagnosis of hypertension.[2-4]

Another disturbing feature of current hypertension management is that even those patients whose blood pressure is satisfactorily controlled remain at a higher risk of cardiovascular complications and death, particularly from coronary heart disease but also from stroke, than normotensive individuals.[5-7] Suboptimal blood pressure control probably contributes to this excess risk, although other factors, such as a history of cigarette smoking, blood cholesterol levels and presence of target organ damage at diagnosis, are important.[7]

Successful hypertension management therefore involves more than simply controlling blood pressure; all cardiovascular risk factors in a patient must be reduced for the patient to benefit fully from treatment. A population approach that ensures healthy lifestyles are promoted to all members of the population is also vital if cardiovascular risk factors are to be reduced.

The pharmacist has an important role to play both in the individual patient with hypertension and as part of the population approach to hypertension management. As indicated above, at the moment many patients with hypertension are not benefiting from their treatment. This is having considerable costs in terms of wasted resources and leaving people at risk of suffering cardiovascular events. Hypertension is a chronic condition that, once diagnosed, probably entails treatment for life. The pharmacist is in an ideal position to provide the necessary support that these patients need for their therapy to be effective. Ensuring patients get the most from their drug therapy is the aim of medicines management or pharmaceutical care – increasingly used phrases in pharmacy practice. Medicines management encompasses: assessment of the prescribed medication; consideration of the therapeutic objectives of the patient and doctor; development of a care plan to resolve and prevent drug therapy problems and to achieve therapeutic goals; and follow-up to evaluate outcomes and review treatment.

Pharmacists are also ideally placed to provide advice on healthy lifestyles and support such as smoking cessation, cholesterol and blood pressure measurement that are necessary for reducing cardiovascular risks in the population as a whole.

These two aspects of the pharmacist's role are recognised in the NHS Plan and expanded in the paper *Pharmacy in the Future – Implementing the NHS Plan*.[8]

The aim of this book is to provide a summary of the information currently available on hypertension management, particularly in relation to drug therapy. It is hoped that this book provides the necessary information to enable pharmacists to provide effective pharmaceutical care of the hypertensive patient. Chapters 2–6 cover the disease and the management of the patient with hypertension and Chapters 7–13 cover the antihypertensive drugs used. Chapter 16 is more specifically directed to the care of the hypertensive patient from the perspective of the pharmacist. This book deals mainly with the patient who has essential or primary hypertension; specialist aspects of hypertension care required during childhood and pregnancy and secondary forms of hypertension are outside the scope of this book. Readers requiring further information on these areas of hypertension management are referred to a list of relevant texts at the end of the book. Any comments or constructive criticisms on the content and layout of the information would be welcome.

Every effort has been made to ensure the accuracy of the information presented in this book, but the rapidly changing nature of much of the information, especially adverse effects and dosage information, should be borne in mind by users. It is recommended that the most recent version of the manufacturer's data sheet or summary of product characteristics be consulted to validate the drug dosage information in particular.

My thanks are due to the library staff of the Royal Pharmaceutical Society for their assistance in providing references and textbooks.

References

1. Prescott-Clarke P, Primatesta T. *Health Service for England 1996. A Survey Carried out on Behalf of the Department of Health.* London: Stationery Office, 1998.
2. Smith W C S, Lee A J, Crombie I K, Tunstall-Pedoe H. Control of blood pressure in Scotland: the rule of halves. *BMJ* 1990; 300: 981–983.
3. Mashru M, Lant A. Interpractice audit of diagnosis and management of hypertension in primary care: educational intervention and review of medical records. *BMJ* 1997; 314: 942–946.
4. Colhoun H M, Dong W, Poulter N R. Blood pressure screening, management and control in England, results from the health survey for England 1994. *J Hypertens* 1998; 16: 747–753.
5. Thürmer H L, Lund-Larsen P G, Tverdal A. Is blood pressure treatment as effective in a population setting as in controlled trials? Results from a prospective study. *J Hypertens* 1994; 12: 481–490.
6. Merlo J, Ranstam J, Liedholm H, *et al.* Incidence of myocardial infarction in elderly men being treated with antihypertensive drugs: population based cohort study. *BMJ* 1996; 313: 457–461.
7. Andersson O K, Almgren T, Persson B, *et al.* Survival in treated hypertension: follow up study after two decades. *BMJ* 1998; 317: 167–171.
8. Department of Health. *Pharmacy in the Future – Implementing the NHS Plan.* London: DoH, 2000.

2

Hypertension

Hypertension is not itself a disease but is a condition of consistently raised blood pressure above 'normal' that, if left untreated, carries a risk of increased morbidity and mortality from various cardiovascular diseases, including stroke and coronary heart disease and renal impairment (see p. 9).

Definition

The term 'blood pressure' refers to the pressure of blood against the blood vessel walls. It generally means arterial blood pressure as it is usually measured indirectly in the brachial artery just above the elbow using a mercury sphygmomanometer (see p. 16) and is expressed in mmHg. Two measurements are made: systolic or maximum blood pressure – the pressure measured during ventricular contraction of the heart – and diastolic or minimum blood pressure – the pressure measured during ventricular dilatation. Blood pressure is therefore usually quoted as two figures, for example, 140/80 mmHg, 140 mmHg being the systolic blood pressure and 80 mmHg being the diastolic blood pressure.

Blood pressure variation within a population

Within a population blood pressure shows a bell-shaped distribution. Thus, there is a continuous range of blood pressures from the lowest to the highest with the majority of individuals falling somewhere in the middle. In most westernised cultures blood pressure increases progressively with age. Sex influences the rise with age. Children have similar blood pressure until teenage years when the blood pressure of boys increases more rapidly so that during early adulthood men have higher blood pressure than women. However, during adulthood the age-related rise in blood pressure is slightly steeper for women so that by the seventh decade of life blood pressure is the same in men and women. Beyond this age, blood pressure increases more quickly in women. The rate of rise of blood pressure with age also appears to be influenced by ethnicity. Blacks tend to have higher blood pressure than whites and the difference increases with increasing age. Some communities worldwide (mostly those that are non-westernised) have low blood pressures and do not show age-related increases. This suggests that lifestyle factors such as diet and exercise are also important determinants of the relation between blood pressure and age.

Just as blood pressures differ in westernised and non-westernised cultures, so there are significant differences in blood pressure within regions of the same country. Alcohol and diet are likely to be important factors in this variation, although it is uncertain how much of the variability they explain.

Genetic component of hypertension

Hypertension tends to cluster within families. While lifestyle habits and shared environment contribute to some of this finding, genetic make-up is also a factor. A very few rare forms of hypertension can be attributed to a single gene mutation. However, the majority of cases of high blood pressure appear to be the result of an interaction of several genes with each other and with the environment. Estimates of the genetic contribution to blood pressure variability range from 30 to 60%. Potential candidate genes include those that affect various components of the renin–angiotensin system, the kallikrein–kinin system and the sympathetic nervous system.

Definition of hypertension or high blood pressure

As blood pressure rises it is associated with various adverse cardiovascular events (see p. 9). This relationship between level of blood pressure and risk of suffering a cardiovascular event (cardiovascular risk) is a continuous one, that is, there is no dividing line between a blood pressure that is free of risk and a blood pressure that represents cardiovascular risk. Blood pressure is also only one of many cardiovascular risk factors. Other factors are listed in Risk Factor Focus (see p. 19). The significance of a particular blood pressure reading will therefore vary from patient to patient. Thus, the definition of normal blood pressure and therefore hypertension is necessarily an arbitrary one.

There are various national and international bodies that produce guidelines on hypertension management and these guidelines propose classifications of different blood pressure levels that are broadly similar (see Diagnostic Focus, p. 7).

Both the Joint National Committee (JNC) guidelines[1] in the US and the World Health Organization/International Society of Hypertension (WHO/ISH) guidelines[2] define an optimal blood pressure with respect to cardiovascular risk as a systolic pressure below 120 mmHg together with a diastolic pressure below 80 mmHg (i.e. <120/<80 mmHg). Normal blood pressure is defined as <130/<85 mmHg and the region between this and 140/90 mmHg is defined as 'high-normal'.

Hypertension is therefore defined as a blood pressure ≥140/≥90 mmHg. Different levels of hypertension are recognised. These are often described as mild, moderate and severe (see Diagnostic Focus, below), although these terms may be misleading in that they do not refer to prognosis since absolute cardiovascular risk, as mentioned above, also depends on other factors. The JNC guidelines[1] use a staging system for classification, while the recent WHO/ISH guidelines[2] prefer to describe them as grades corresponding to their previous descriptions of mild, moderate and severe. The British Hypertension Society (BHS) guidelines[3] have moved away from such firm categories with the increasing recognition of the influence of other cardiovascular risk factors on treatment decisions but they generally recognise similar degrees of hypertension.

Note that when the systolic and diastolic pressure fall into different categories, the higher grade or stage is used for classification purposes.

DIAGNOSTIC FOCUS

Definitions of 'normal' blood pressure and hypertension (in mmHg)					
Optimal	Normal	High-normal	Grade 1/ stage 1 hypertension (mild)	Grade 2/ stage 2 hypertension (moderate)	Grade 3/ stage 3 hypertension (severe)
<120/ <80	<130/ <85	130–139/ 85–89	140–159/ 90–99 Subgroup: borderline 140–149/ 90–94	160–179/ 100–109	≥180/ ≥110

NB: Where systolic and diastolic blood pressure fall into different categories, the higher grade/stage is used for classification purposes. For example, a blood pressure of 135/90 mmHg places the patient in grade 1/stage 1.

Isolated systolic hypertension

Diastolic blood pressure tends to plateau before the age of 60 years and drop thereafter. The drop in diastolic blood pressure occurs because of the loss of distensibility and elasticity in the large-capacitance arteries and this is a reflection of widespread atherosclerosis. Since systolic blood pressure continues to rise progressively this produces a situation where the diastolic blood pressure is within normal limits but the systolic pressure is higher than normal. This is referred to as isolated systolic hypertension and occurs mainly in the elderly. It has been defined as systolic pressure of 160 mmHg or more[3] (or 140 mmHg or more[1,2]) and diastolic pressure under 90 mmHg (see Diagnostic Focus, below). The WHO/ISH[2] also recognise a subgroup they define as borderline isolated systolic hypertension of 140–149/<90 mmHg.

DIAGNOSTIC FOCUS

Isolated systolic hypertension	
Systolic pressure (mmHg)	Diastolic pressure (mmHg)
≥160* or ≥140†	<90
*BHS guidelines.[3] †JNC[1] and WHO/ISH guidelines.[2]	

Causes

In the majority of cases of hypertension (over 95%) there is no immediately obvious underlying cause; such cases are referred to as primary or essential hypertension. It is suspected that such primary or essential hypertension is multifactorial in origin, with various factors such as environmental influences, diet and body weight playing a role. Genetic factors are also thought to contribute since hypertension clusters in families (see p. 6).

In a small minority of patients (2–5% of hypertensives), hypertension is due to an underlying disease, usually involving the kidneys or endocrine system (see Risk Factor Focus, p. 9), or may be due to the adverse effects of drugs (see Risk Factor Focus, p. 9). Such hypertension is referred to as secondary hypertension. Secondary hypertension may be suspected particularly in resistant or malignant hypertension. Effective treatment of the underlying condition can sometimes, but not necessarily, abolish the hypertension.

RISK FACTOR FOCUS

Some causes of secondary hypertension

- Endocrine, including phaeochromocytoma, Conn's syndrome, Cushing's syndrome, hyperparathyroidism, acromegaly
- Renal, including renal parenchymal disease (such as glomerulonephritis, polycystic diseases), renovascular hypertension, renin-producing tumours
- Coarctation of the aorta
- Neurological disorders, including sleep apnoea, brain tumours, Guillain–Barré syndrome
- Drugs (see Risk Factor Focus below)
- Pregnancy – pre-eclampsia
- Surgery

RISK FACTOR FOCUS

Drugs that can cause hypertension

Alcohol (chronic consumption)
Amphetamines
Anorectics
Caffeine
Carbenoxolone
Ciclosporin
Cocaine
Corticosteroids
Ergot alkaloids
Erythropoietin
Herbal remedies containing bayberry, broom, capsicum, blue cohosh, cola, coltsfoot, gentian, ginger, panax ginseng, liquorice, mate, vervain
Nicotine
Non-steroidal anti-inflammatory drugs
Oral contraceptives
Sympathomimetics
Venlafaxine

Consequences of hypertension

Untreated hypertension can lead to the development of various cardio-vascular or cerebrovascular disorders and renal effects, outlined below. Such effects are sometimes referred to as target organ damage. Hyper-tension may be the sole contributory factor in the development of some of the conditions while other disorders have more complex origins, with hypertension being only one of many contributory factors. The extent of organ damage often correlates with the level of blood pressure, although this is not always the case. Sometimes markedly high pressures are seen with no evidence of target organ damage and, conversely, organ damage may be present with only moderate elevation of blood pressure. There is also marked variation between individuals in the rate of progression of target organ damage. Many factors, which are at present poorly understood, probably influence the rate of progression. Whatever the level of blood pressure, the presence of organ damage increases the risks of cardiovascular complications occurring.

Stroke

One of the most devastating consequences of hypertension is stroke; it results not only in premature death but also in significant disability. Elderly patients with hypertension are particularly prone to all forms of stroke and often sustain multiple short episodes of cerebral ischaemia (transient ischaemic attacks) that lead to progressive loss of intellectual function and dementia.

In patients with hypertension, about 80% of strokes are ischaemic, caused by intra-arterial thrombosis or embolisation from the heart and large arteries. The remaining 20% are from haemorrhagic causes. Hypertension is the most important modifiable risk factor for stroke and transient ischaemic attacks. In the UK it is estimated that 40% of all strokes are attributable to a systolic blood pressure of 140 mmHg or more. Blood pressure levels have been shown to be positively and continuously related to the risk of stroke (both haemorrhagic and ischaemic) across a wide range of levels. The positive association appears to be steeper for haemorrhagic stroke than ischaemic stroke. Hypertension is also associated with an increased risk of atrial fibrillation that also contributes to an increased stroke risk.

Population studies indicate that an average reduction in diastolic blood pressure of just 5 mmHg produces a 35–40% reduction in risk of stroke.[4,5] No lower level has been identified below which the risk of stroke did not continue to decline. A recent study of the treatment of elderly patients (>60 years of age) with isolated systolic hypertension has also shown that dementia can be prevented by lowering high blood pressure.[6]

Coronary heart disease

Fatal coronary heart disease is the major population consequence of hypertension; it is seven times more common among patients with hypertension than fatal stroke. Blood pressure levels have been shown to be continuously and positively related to the risk of developing coronary heart disease (angina, myocardial infarction or sudden death), although the strength of this association is about two-thirds as steep as that for stroke. This weaker association between blood pressure level and risk of coronary heart disease is a reflection of the importance of other risk factors in addition to hypertension in the development of coronary heart disease. The relatively greater importance of other risk factors means that the reduction in coronary heart disease seen in trials of blood pressure lowering is much less impressive than the effect on stroke and heart failure. Nevertheless, analysis of the large treatment trials (based on blood pressure reduction with thiazides and beta blockers) suggests that adequate treatment of hypertension reduces the risk of myocardial infarction by approximately 20%.

Heart failure

Heart failure has a poor long-term prognosis. The precise relationship between blood pressure level and risk of heart failure is not as clearly established as that for stroke and coronary heart disease. Nevertheless, evidence from prospective epidemiological studies suggests that patients with a history of hypertension have at least a six times greater risk of heart failure than do individuals without such a history. Data suggest that antihypertensive treatment, although not completely preventing heart failure, can postpone the development of heart failure by several decades.

Left ventricular hypertrophy

Left ventricular hypertrophy (increased mass of left ventricular muscle) occurs as a compensatory response to the increased afterload imposed on the heart by high blood pressure. Eventually the increased muscle mass outstrips its oxygen supply and this, coupled with the reduced coronary vascular reserve seen in hypertension, can result in myocardial ischaemia even with normal coronary arteries. Left ventricular hypertrophy secondary to hypertension is a major risk factor for myocardial infarction, stroke, sudden death and heart failure. Hypertensives with left ventricular hypertrophy are also at increased risk of cardiac arrhythmias (atrial fibrillation and ventricular arrhythmias) and atherosclerotic vascular disease (coronary and peripheral artery disease).

The development of echocardiography has shown that the incidence of left ventricular hypertrophy is considerably higher than previously realised and is commonly found in mild hypertension. These findings have focused attention on the effectiveness of the different classes of antihypertensive drug in causing regression of left ventricular hypertrophy.

Vascular diseases

Vascular diseases include abdominal aortic aneurysm and peripheral vascular disease. Development of these diseases reflects generalised atherosclerosis that is exacerbated by hypertension. Intermittent claudication, which is a manifestation of peripheral vascular disease, is about three times more common in patients with hypertension. Many patients with peripheral vascular disease also have renal artery stenosis, which may be contributing to their hypertension.

Hypertension also increases the incidence of atherosclerotic lesions in the carotid arteries. Severe carotid artery stenosis is known to be a frequent cause of stroke and ulcerated plaques can be a source of emboli provoking ischaemic strokes or transient ischaemic attacks.

Renal disease

The risk of renal disease is related to blood pressure levels, although the size of the relationship is less well established than that for stroke or coronary heart disease. Renal involvement varies from asymptomatic through to renal failure. The first objective sign of renal damage is microalbuminuria, which is often demonstrable in patients with only minimally raised blood pressures. The presence of microalbuminuria is a predictor of progressive renal damage and of overall cardiovascular morbidity. Some patients with hypertension and renal damage go on to develop renal failure. However, there is some controversy as to whether patients with mild-to-moderate essential hypertension can go on to develop renal failure. Some consider that those who do eventually develop renal failure in fact have hypertension secondary to renal disease. Malignant hypertension frequently leads to progressive renal failure.

Retinopathy

Hypertension leads to various vascular changes in the eye, referred to as hypertensive retinopathy. The changes may include bilateral retinal flame-shaped haemorrhages, cotton wool spots, hard exudates and papilloedema.

Detection of patients with hypertension

Hypertension may only be detected once symptoms of target organ damage appear. However, more often hypertension is asymptomatic and is discovered during routine blood pressure measurement. The importance of regular blood pressure measurement is discussed in Chapter 15, on primary prevention and screening.

References

1. Joint National Committee. The sixth report of the Joint National Committee on prevention, detection, evaluation, and treatment of high blood pressure (JNC VI). *Arch Intern Med* 1997; 157: 2413–2446. Correction *ibid*. 1998; 158: 573.
2. Guidelines Subcommittee. 1999 World Health Organization–International Society of Hypertension guidelines for the management of hypertension. *J Hypertens* 1999; 17: 151–183.
3. Ramsay L E, Williams B, Johnston G D, *et al*. BHS guidelines. Guidelines for management of hypertension: report of the third working party of the British Hypertension Society. *J Hum Hypertens* 1999; 13: 569–592.
4. Eastern Stroke and Coronary Heart Disease Collaborative Research Group. Blood pressure, cholesterol, and stroke in eastern Asia. *Lancet* 1998; 352: 1801–1807.
5. MacMahon S, Peto R, Cutler J, *et al*. Blood pressure, stroke, and coronary heart disease. Part 1, prolonged differences in blood pressure: prospective observational studies corrected for the regression dilution bias. *Lancet* 1990; 335: 765–774.
6. Forette F, Seux M-L, Staessen J A, *et al*. Prevention of dementia in randomised double-blind placebo-controlled systolic hypertension in Europe (Syst-Eur) trial. *Lancet* 1998; 352: 1347–1351.

3

Hypertension management

The management of hypertension can be divided into a population approach and an individual approach. The population approach involves implementing measures that aim to reduce the blood pressure in the entire population and thus prevent the development of complications of hypertension (see Chapter 15, on primary prevention and screening). The individual approach involves treating those patients found to have elevated blood pressure either because they have symptoms or suffer a cardiovascular event or, more commonly, at routine screening.

This chapter focuses on the treatment of individual patients (adults) with primary or essential hypertension. The management of hypertensive crises, or hypertension in children, in patients with renal disease, in pregnancy, or in surgery is outside the scope of this book. General textbooks on hypertension that include the management of these patient groups and more specific references can be found in the recommended reading section at the end of the book.

The management of hypertension involves the following:

- Confirmation of diagnosis, including blood pressure measurement
- Patient assessment
- Treatment options
- Selection of whom to treat with drugs
- Treatment goals
- Management of contributory conditions
- Follow-up.

Confirmation of diagnosis

A single blood pressure reading cannot be used to diagnose a patient as being hypertensive. The measurement of blood pressure (see below for technique) is recognised as being a very inaccurate procedure and within an individual patient blood pressure can vary considerably, both at repeated measurements at a single visit and on separate occasions. Some of the reasons for blood pressure variation are given in Diagnostic Focus (see below). One of the most important aspects of the management of a patient presenting with high blood pressure is therefore to confirm the diagnosis of hypertension by taking repeated blood pressure measurements before the patient is started on what could be lifelong antihypertensive therapy. When an average is taken of several blood pressure readings over a period of time, a significant number of patients may be able to be reclassified as normotensive. The length of the observation period with re-measurement depends on the severity of the hypertension. In severe hypertension, prolonged observation before treatment will not be needed. However, in patients with mild-to-moderate hypertension the British Hypertension Society (BHS) guidelines recommend an average of two readings per visit at monthly intervals for 4–6 months to guide treatment decisions.[1]

DIAGNOSTIC FOCUS

Factors producing variation in blood pressure readings
<ul><li>Measurer's technique</li><li>Time of day – blood pressure tends to be highest first thing in the morning and lowest at night</li><li>Temperature – cold temperature increases blood pressure (keep the room used for measurement at a reasonable temperature)</li><li>Obesity – a falsely high reading will be given if too small a cuff is used</li><li>Anxiety increases blood pressure (discuss test with patient)</li><li>Full bladder increases blood pressure</li><li>Tight clothing increases blood pressure</li><li>Consumption of caffeine, tobacco or alcohol increases blood pressure</li></ul>

Blood pressure measurement

Major changes are now underway in this most commonly performed procedure. A mercury sphygmomanometer has been the gold standard for routine clinical practice for many years, but for health and safety reasons the use of mercury is declining and will eventually cease completely. In the future there will be increasing use of alternative methods such as aneroid, semiautomated and automated devices; many such devices are now available, but few have been independently evaluated for accuracy. This is especially true of devices for self-measurement. The European Society of Hypertension has undertaken to review blood pressure measuring devices regularly to determine which devices may be recommended.[2] Whatever device is used, regular maintenance and calibration are important. Frequent retraining and meticulous technique of the person performing the measurement are also vital in ensuring the accuracy of the procedure.

The BHS recommendations should be followed when measuring a patient's blood pressure.[3] The patient should be seated in a quiet room with the arm supported at the same level as the heart. Tight clothing should be removed and the hand should be relaxed. When taking blood pressure using a sphygmomanometer, it is important that the correct size of cuff is used. The air bladder of the cuff should encircle at least three-quarters and preferably the whole of the upper arm; the use of too small a cuff will result in an overestimation of the blood pressure. The cuff should be inflated to about 20 mmHg above the systolic pressure as indicated by the disappearance of the radial pulse. It should then be deflated at 2 mmHg/s and the systolic pressure recorded at the first appearance of the auscultatory sounds. The diastolic pressure is indicated by the disappearance of these sounds. Two measurements should be taken on each visit. Seated blood pressure readings are generally sufficient, but standing blood pressure should also be measured in elderly patients, those with diabetes, or other conditions where orthostatic hypotension is common. Blood pressure should be measured in both arms if peripheral vascular disease is evident or suspected.

'White coat' hypertension

Some patients develop high blood pressure when their blood pressure is taken by doctors in a hospital or clinic environment – the so-called 'white coat' effect. 'White coat' hypertension should be suspected in patients who have persistently elevated blood pressures when measured in a clinic environment but little or no evidence of target organ damage. It should also be suspected in patients who develop symptoms of hypotension even with small doses of antihypertensive drugs. Home blood pressure measurements with an automated device or 24-hour ambulatory blood pressure monitoring will confirm the diagnosis of 'white coat' hypertension in these cases.

Ambulatory and home blood pressure monitoring

Ambulatory blood pressure monitoring provides numerous readings over a short time and therefore reduces variability compared with the average of a limited number of surgery readings. In addition to its use in diagnosing 'white coat' hypertension, it may also be used when blood pressure shows unusual variability, in hypertension which is resistant to drug therapy, or when symptoms suggest the possibility of hypotension while on medication. It may also be useful in patients with episodic hypertension or autonomic dysfunction.

Self-measurement of blood pressure at home is an alternative to ambulatory blood pressure monitoring: it is more convenient for the patient and less expensive. It can be used to monitor response to treatment and to ensure that there is adequate blood pressure control during the day. It is also useful as an aid to improving patient compliance.

It is important to note that home and ambulatory blood pressure readings are usually a few mmHg lower than clinic readings. Most guidelines and recommendations are based on clinic blood pressure readings.

Patient assessment

Each new patient requires a thorough clinical assessment, one of the primary aims of which is to exclude a secondary cause of the hypertension. Although secondary causes account for fewer than 5% of hypertension cases, they are important to identify, as they are often either correctable or represent serious underlying disease. The majority of secondary causes are renal, endocrine or due to concomitant contraceptive pills or non-steroidal anti-inflammatory drugs (see Chapter 2 for more details of secondary causes). The clinical assessment also aims to identify any complications of hypertension (see p. 9) and any cardiovascular risk factors or contributory factors (see Risk Factor Focus, p. 19). Any concomitant conditions that will influence choice of drug or prognosis should also be looked for, as well as any contraindications to the major groups of antihypertensive drugs.

The clinical assessment should include a full physical examination and full history. There are only a few routine investigations that are needed and these should include:

- Urine strip test for protein/blood
- Serum creatinine and electrolytes
- Blood glucose
- Serum total: high-density lipoprotein cholesterol ratio
- Electrocardiogram.

In some individuals, the clinical evaluation or results of these simple investigations will suggest a need for further investigations, such as echocardiogram or renal ultrasound.

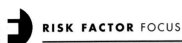

RISK FACTOR FOCUS

Factors influencing cardiovascular risk

Risk factors
Smoking
Diabetes
Total cholesterol: high-density lipoprotein cholesterol ratio (dyslipidaemia)
Family history of premature cardiovascular disease: women <65 years, men <55 years
Age
Sex (male gender – a lower level of risk is seen in women at least until age 55)
Postmenopausal status

Target organ disease
Previous cardiovascular events/overt cardiovascular disease

- Angina
- Heart failure
- Coronary revascularisation (percutaneous transluminal angioplasty, coronary artery bypass graft)
- Myocardial infarction
- Stroke
- Transient ischaemic attack

Left ventricular hypertrophy
Peripheral vascular disease
Proteinuria
Renal impairment
Retinopathy
Atherosclerotic plaque in aorta, carotid, iliac or femoral arteries

Contributory factors
Obesity
Sedentary lifestyle
Excess alcohol intake

In general, more aggressive investigation is called for when the patient is younger or the hypertension is more severe.

Treatment options

Lifestyle measures and drug therapy are the two methods used to reduce blood pressure. All patients should be given advice on lifestyle measures to adopt that will reduce their blood pressure and cardiovascular risk factors (see Chapter 6 for more details). In some patients lifestyle measures may produce a sufficient fall in blood pressure on their own and patients with only mildly elevated blood pressures should be given a trial of several weeks before deciding whether to add in drug therapy (see Management Focus, p. 22, on thresholds for treatment). Patients with higher blood pressure will need drug treatment in addition to lifestyle measures. The choice of drug should be made on an individual basis and this process is discussed in Chapter 4.

In addition to these measures of reducing blood pressure, it is important that measures are taken to reduce any other cardiovascular risk factors or contributory conditions that are present (see p. 24).

Selection of whom to treat with drugs

Much of the discussion of hypertension management centres on when to intervene with drugs in those patients whose blood pressure is only mildly raised. The decision to use drug treatment is clear-cut in patients whose blood pressure is markedly raised, for example, patients whose blood pressure is >160/100 mmHg. These patients are individually at greatest risk of stroke and coronary heart disease and clearly require drug treatment to reduce their blood pressure (choice of agent is discussed in Chapter 4). However, patients with very high blood pressure like this form only a small group of those with hypertension and even if they all had their blood pressure perfectly controlled it would have little impact on the total number of strokes or heart attacks occurring in the population as a whole.

The majority of patients with hypertension have blood pressures in the range 140–159/90–99 mmHg – so-called mild hypertension. It is amongst these patients that the majority of cardiovascular events occur. For example, prospective observational studies indicate that 80% of coronary events and 70% of strokes occur in individuals with a usual systolic blood pressure below 155 mmHg and a diastolic blood pressure below 95 mmHg. However, if all these people were to be assigned to drug treatment, the costs would be enormous. In addition, since these patients are usually asymptomatic, the use of drugs, probably for life, with potential adverse effects needs very careful consideration.

The main clinical problem, then, is which of these patients with mild hypertension should be given drug treatment.

Over the years it has become clear that decisions about the management of a patient with mild hypertension cannot be made solely on the patient's blood pressure reading. This is because hypertension is only one of several factors that increase the risk of a patient suffering a cardio-vascular or cerebrovascular event. Important factors that predict cardio-vascular risk are listed in Risk Factor Focus (see p. 19). The most powerful predictor of future risk of cardiovascular events in the patient with hypertension is pre-existing cardiovascular disease. Diabetes and evidence of other hypertensive target organ damage, such as left ven-tricular hypertrophy, proteinuria or severe retinopathy, are also import-ant predictors of future risk. The risk of developing cardiovascular disease can therefore range from low to high in patients with mild hyper-tension depending on whether, or what, other associated risk factors are present. For example, a 65-year-old male smoker with a blood pressure of 145/90 mmHg who has a history of transient ischaemic attacks and diabetes has an annual risk of a major cardiovascular event which is more than 20 times greater than that in a 40-year-old man with the same blood pressure but no history of transient ischaemic attacks or diabetes.

Current guidelines therefore recommend that the overall cardio-vascular risk of the patient with mild hypertension must be considered before a decision about drug treatment can be made. Patients with mild hypertension (140–159/90–99 mmHg) who have diabetes, existing cardiovascular disease or other target organ damage are at sufficiently high risk of suffering a future cardiovascular event to require drug treat-ment. In patients with mild hypertension without these additional factors an estimate of their cardiovascular risk is needed before a decision about drug treatment can be made.

A problem in the past has been making an accurate estimate of a patient's cardiovascular risk when no formal method was recommended. Several algorithms and computer programs are now available that allow accurate estimation of cardiovascular risk by counting the major risk factors and weighting them using risk functions derived from epidemio-logical studies. The BHS guidelines[1] recommend that one of these com-puter programs, the 'cardiac risk assessor' and a coronary heart disease risk chart based on the Framingham risk function, be used to estimate 10-year coronary heart disease risk. (The coronary risk prediction chart is reproduced in the *British National Formulary*.[4]) If the patient's 10-year coronary heart disease risk is ≥15%, then antihypertensive drug treatment is recommended. This method of formal estimation of coron-ary heart disease risk is also used to aid decision making in the treat-ment of hypertensives with aspirin or statins (see p. 24).

Both the World Health Organization/International Society of Hypertension (WHO/ISH) guidelines[5] and the Joint National Commit-tee (JNC) guidelines[6] use an approach that divides patients into three or four risk categories on the basis of their blood pressure, cardiovascular risk factors, target organ damage and associated clinical conditions (such as cardiovascular or renal disease).

Management Focus (see below) summarises the current BHS guidelines for intervention with drugs in patients with hypertension, which are broadly in line with the JNC and WHO/ISH guidelines.

Treatment goals

Undertreatment of patients with hypertension is a significant problem (see Chapter 1). To make sure that patients obtain the necessary benefit

MANAGEMENT FOCUS

Thresholds for treatment		
Blood pressure (mmHg)	Additional factors*	Action
≥220/120		Immediate drug treatment. Advise on lifestyle measures (see Chapter 6)
200–219/110–119		Confirm over 1–2 weeks, then start drug treatment. Advise on lifestyle measures
160–199/100–109	Yes	Confirm over 3–4 weeks, then start drug treatment. Advise on lifestyle measures
	No	Advise on lifestyle measures. Re-measure blood pressure weekly; start drug treatment if blood pressure persists over 4–12 weeks
140–159/90–99	Yes	Advise on lifestyle measures. Confirm blood pressure over weeks, then start drug treatment
	No	Advise on lifestyle measures. Re-measure blood pressure monthly. If blood pressure persists, estimate CHD risk and start drug treatment if 10-year CHD risk ≥15%. If risk <15%, reassess yearly
135–139/85–89		Reassess yearly
<135/85		Reassess in 5 years

*Existing cardiovascular disease, diabetes or target organ damage.
CHD = Coronary heart disease.

from their treatment, it is vital that the goals of treatment are clearly established from the outset. Having clear aims can also aid patient compliance with treatment (see Chapter 16). The goal of treatment must be to prevent the complications of hypertension by reducing blood pressure to as near normal levels as possible (see below) and to detect and correct other cardiovascular risk factors. This should be achieved, as far as possible, without causing the patient adverse effects from medication or other interventions.

Target blood pressure

There has been concern in the past that the over-aggressive reduction of diastolic pressure might increase the risk of ischaemic heart disease (the so-called J-curve effect). However, the HOT study[7] that looked at blood pressure levels achieved during therapy has produced clearer guidance over target blood pressures and in particular has provided reassurance that reducing diastolic blood pressure to <80 mmHg does not increase cardiovascular risk. The study assigned hypertensive patients to three different target diastolic blood pressures (≤90, ≤85 or ≤80 mmHg). The difference in blood pressures between the different target groups ended up being only about 2 mmHg, and this narrow blood pressure difference was too small to translate into any significant difference in cardiovascular outcomes between the groups. However, the study did show that those assigned to the lowest blood pressure target did not suffer any untoward effects and subgroup analysis of patients with diabetes found that lowering blood pressure to the lowest target pressure produced a significant reduction in cardiovascular events. This finding is consistent with results from the UK Prospective Diabetes Study Group.[8] This study found that diabetic patients with hypertension assigned to tight blood pressure control (whose blood pressure averaged 144/82 mmHg) had a lower risk of cardiovascular events compared with diabetic patients not assigned to tight control and whose average blood pressure was 154/87 mmHg.

Current guidelines vary slightly in their recommended target blood pressures, although they all reflect the need for patients with diabetes in particular to achieve lower blood pressures. The guidelines also recognise that the lower blood pressures may be difficult to achieve in practice and therefore in addition to citing an optimal blood pressure to aim for, they also include a higher blood pressure target that should be the aim in those patients who fail to attain the optimal blood pressure (i.e. a minimum recommended goal). The JNC guidelines[6] cite an optimal blood pressure of <120/80 mmHg, and <140/90 mmHg as a minimum target. BHS guidelines[1] recommend an optimal blood pressure target of <140/85 mmHg, with a blood pressure of at least <150/90 mmHg being reached. In patients with diabetes the optimal target is <140/80 mmHg with a minimum target of <140/85 mmHg. The BHS guidelines[1] also stress the importance of both systolic and diastolic blood pressures reaching the target pressures. WHO/ISH[5] suggest <130/85 mmHg as the blood pressure goal for young or middle-aged patients or those with diabetes and <140/90 mmHg for elderly patients. These recommendations are for clinic measurements. If home or ambulatory blood pressure measurements are being used to monitor treatment then it should be remembered that blood pressures would be lower by an average of 10–15 mmHg systolic and 5–10 mmHg diastolic.

It is essential that regular review be undertaken to ensure that the target blood pressures are achieved and maintained in the long term.

Management of contributory conditions

Despite the benefits of blood pressure lowering treatment established in randomised controlled trials, several population studies have demonstrated that treated hypertensive patients continue to experience substantially higher risks of coronary heart disease, stroke and overall mortality than do non-hypertensive individuals some years after beginning antihypertensive drug therapy.[9–13] There are many possible reasons for this persisting excess risk. Undertreatment undoubtedly contributes, as does failure to control other cardiovascular risk factors in a patient. Therefore successful treatment of hypertension involves not only controlling blood pressure adequately but ensuring that all other risk factors and contributory conditions such as diabetes are adequately treated as well. Thorough patient assessment is therefore important to determine other risk factors. Lifestyle measures (see Chapter 6) will control some of the risk factors, but patients should also be assessed to see whether they would benefit from aspirin therapy or lipid lowering therapy with statins.

Antiplatelet therapy

The benefits of long-term therapy with aspirin and some other antiplatelet agents are well established in patients with a history of coronary heart disease or cerebrovascular disease; the risks of fatal and non-fatal coronary events, stroke and cardiovascular death are all reduced. The BHS guidelines[1] recommend that aspirin 75 mg daily should be given to hypertensive patients with cardiovascular complications.

In patients without a history of cardiovascular disease the benefits are less clear. Studies such as the Antiplatelet Trialists' Collaboration,[14] HOT[7] and the Thrombosis Prevention Trial[15] have shown reduction in risks of coronary heart disease but no clear reduction in stroke or total cardiovascular death. In these studies there has been an increase in non-cerebral bleeding risks. For primary prevention, therefore, the benefits in reduction of coronary heart disease must be balanced against the bleeding risks.

The BHS guidelines[1] recommend that aspirin 75 mg daily should be given to those patients aged ≥50 years who have satisfactory control of their blood pressure and who have evidence of target organ damage (left ventricular hypertrophy, proteinuria or renal impairment), type 2 diabetes or a 10-year coronary heart disease risk ≥15%.

Statins

Cholesterol lowering with statins (HMG CoA reductase inhibitors) has been shown to reduce the risks of coronary heart disease events (fatal and non-fatal) in both primary and secondary prevention studies.[16–19] Reductions in stroke risk have also been observed in patients with coronary heart disease.[18] In the few trials that provided data on cerebral infarction, there was some evidence of reduction in the risk of this stroke subtype. Hypertensive patients included in these studies showed similar benefits to the overall findings on subgroup analysis.[18,19] The persistent risk of coronary and stroke death in treated hypertensive patients has been linked among other factors to serum cholesterol concentrations before and during treatment. Therefore statins should be used in patients with elevated cholesterol levels.

BHS guidelines[1] recommend targeting statin therapy at those at highest cardiovascular risk: serum total cholesterol ≥5 mmol/l and existing cardiovascular disease or 10-year coronary heart disease risk ≥30% (estimated using the Joint British Societies cardiac risk assessor programme[1] or risk chart). Statins are also recommended for those with familial hypercholesterolaemia. The upper age limits for starting statin therapy are 75 years for secondary prevention and 70 years for primary prevention.

Follow-up

Patients who are treated with drugs need frequent follow-up in the initial stages as drug treatment is titrated to achieve the target blood pressure (see p. 37). Once the target blood pressure is reached and the patient is stabilised on a drug regimen, regular follow-up is still needed to ensure that target blood pressures are maintained, to monitor for drug side-effects and to assess patient compliance with the drug treatment and life-style measures. The frequency of this follow-up should be determined individually, taking into account factors such as severity of the hyper-tension, overall cardiovascular risk, variability of blood pressure and patient compliance with drug and lifestyle regimens. Review every 3 months is sufficient when treatment and blood pressure are stable; the interval should not generally exceed 6 months.

Follow-up is still important in the management of the patient with mild hypertension for whom drug treatment has not been deemed neces-sary. It is essential to continue observation and monitoring of blood pres-sure in these patients at least once a year, since in about 10–15% of these patients blood pressure will rise within 5 years to levels clearly requir-ing treatment.[20] In addition coronary heart disease risk will increase with age, and risk should be reassessed at yearly intervals. These patients should all be encouraged to continue with lifestyle measures to lower blood pressure and cardiovascular risk (see Chapter 6). See Management Focus (p. 27) for a summary of management stages in hypertension.

Withdrawal of drug treatment

Once a patient starts drug treatment for hypertension it is generally the case that this treatment will be lifelong. However, there have been some reports of successful withdrawal in selected patients.[21,22] The JNC guide-lines[6] in the US suggest that patients with mild hypertension with no target organ damage whose blood pressure has been effectively con-trolled for at least a year may be candidates for a reduction in the dosage and number of drugs. The WHO/ISH guidelines[5] also suggest that reduc-tion in antihypertensive therapy may be successful in well-controlled patients. The reduction in antihypertensive drug(s) must be very gradual, with close monitoring of blood pressure. In some patients, particularly those who adhere closely to lifestyle measures, complete withdrawal of antihypertensive treatment might be possible. However, it should be stressed that, even if complete withdrawal is achieved, blood pressure

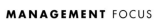

MANAGEMENT FOCUS

Stages of management of the patient with hypertension

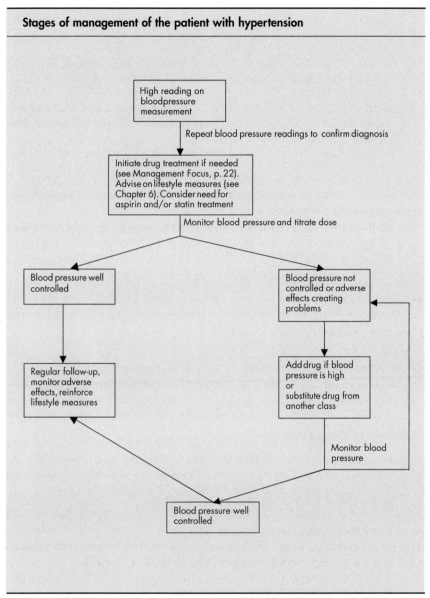

needs to be monitored indefinitely as blood pressure usually rises again sometimes months or even years after discontinuation. The importance of continuing lifestyle measures in these patients should be emphasised.

References

1. Ramsay L E, Williams B, Johnston G D, *et al*. BHS guidelines. Guidelines for management of hypertension: report of the third working party of the British Hypertension Society. *J Hum Hypertens* 1999; 13: 569–592.

2. O'Brien E, Waeber B, Parati G, *et al*. Blood pressure measuring devices: recommendations of the European Society of Hypertension. *BMJ* 2001; 322: 531–536.

3. O'Brien E T, Petrie J C, Littler W A *et al*. *Blood Pressure Measurement: Recommendations of the British Hypertension Society*, 3rd edn. London: BMJ Publishing Group, 1997.

4. Mehta D K, ed. *British National Formulary*, no. 40. London: British Medical Association/RPSGB, 2000.

5. Guidelines Subcommittee. 1999 World Health Organization–International Society of Hypertension guidelines for the management of hypertension. *J Hypertens* 1999; 17: 151–183.

6. Joint National Committee. The sixth report of the Joint National Committee on prevention, detection, evaluation, and treatment of high blood pressure (JNC VI). *Arch Intern Med* 1997; 157: 2413–2446. Correction *ibid*. 1998; 158: 573.

7. Hansson L, Zanchetti A, Carruthers S G, *et al*. Effects of intensive blood-pressure lowering and low-dose aspirin in patients with hypertension: principal results of the Hypertension Optimal Treatment (HOT) randomised trial. *Lancet* 1998; 351: 1755–1762.

8. UK Prospective Diabetes Study Group. Tight blood pressure control and risk of macrovascular and microvascular complications in type 2 diabetes: UKPDS 38. *BMJ* 1998; 317: 703–713. Correction *ibid*. 1999; 318: 29.

9. Collins R, Peto R, MacMahon S, *et al*. Blood pressure, stroke, and coronary heart disease. Part 2, short-term reductions in blood pressure: overview of randomised drug trials in their epidemiological context. *Lancet* 1990; 335: 827–838.

10. Isles C G, Walker L M, Beevers G D, *et al*. Mortality in patients of the Glasgow blood pressure clinic. *J Hypertens* 1986; 4: 141–156.

11. Clausen J, Jenson G. Blood pressure and mortality: an epidemiological survey with 10 years follow-up. *J Hum Hypertens* 1992; 6: 53–59.

12. Merlo J, Ranstam J, Liedholm H, *et al*. Incidence of myocardial infarction in elderly men being treated with antihypertensive drugs: population based cohort study. *BMJ* 1996; 313: 457–461.

13. Andersson O K, Almgren T, Persson B, *et al*. Survival in treated hypertension: follow-up study after two decades. *BMJ* 1998; 317: 167–171.

14. Antiplatelet Trialists' Collaboration. Collaborative overview of randomised trials of antiplatelet therapy – I: prevention of death, myocardial infarction, and stroke by prolonged antiplatelet therapy in various categories of patients. *BMJ* 1994; 308: 81–106. Correction *ibid*.: 1540.

15. The Medical Research Council's General Practice Research Framework. Thrombosis prevention trial: randomised trial of low-intensity oral anti-coagulation with warfarin and low-dose aspirin in the primary prevention of ischaemic heart disease in men at increased risk. *Lancet* 1998; 351: 233–241.

16. Scandinavian Simvastatin Survival Study Group. Randomised trial of cholesterol lowering in 4444 patients with coronary heart disease: the Scandinavian Simvastatin Survival Study (4S). *Lancet* 1994; 344: 1383–1389.

17. Shepherd J, Cobbe S M, Ford I, *et al*. Prevention of coronary heart disease with pravastatin in men with hypercholesterolemia. *N Engl J Med* 1995; 333: 1301–1307.

18. Sacks F M, Pfeffer M A, Moye L A, *et al*. The effect of pravastatin on coronary events after myocardial infarction in patients with average cholesterol levels. *N Engl J Med* 1996; 335: 1001–1009.

19. Downs J R, Clearfield M, Weis S, *et al*. Primary prevention of acute coronary events with lovastatin in men and women with average cholesterol levels: results of AFCAPS/TexCAPS. *JAMA* 1998; 279: 1615–1622.

20. Moser M, Hebert P R. Prevention of disease progression, left ventricular hypertrophy and congestive heart failure in hypertension treatment trials. *J Am Coll Cardiol* 1996; 27: 1214–1218.

21. van den Bosch W J H M, Mol W, van Gerwen W, Thien T. Withdrawal of antihypertensive drugs in selected patients. *Lancet* 1994; 343: 1157.

22. Aylett M J, Creighton P, Jachuck S, *et al*. Withdrawing antihypertensive drugs. *Lancet* 1994; 343: 1512.

4

Pharmacotherapeutic interventions with antihypertensive drugs

Once it has been decided that a patient should be started on an anti-hypertensive drug, which one should be used? The number of classes of antihypertensive drugs has grown considerably over the last 40 years and there are now many different classes to choose from. In the past a widely used approach to drug use in hypertension was the 'stepped-care' approach, which entailed a diuretic or beta blocker as step 1, a diuretic with a beta blocker as step 2, and addition of (usually) a vasodilator as step 3. However, this approach could mean that a patient might be taking three drugs, none of which was providing adequate response, with increased risk of adverse effects. The last 10 years or so have seen the philosophy of drug choice move away from this rigid model. Current guidelines recommend that drug choice should be individualised for each patient, taking into account any concomitant disease and risk factors when deciding on the most appropriate therapy.

Comparing the different classes of antihypertensive drug

The six main antihypertensive drug groups are:

- Thiazides and related diuretics (see Chapter 7)
- Beta blockers (see Chapter 8)
- Angiotensin-converting enzyme (ACE) inhibitors (see Chapter 9)
- Calcium-channel blockers (see Chapter 10)
- Alpha blockers (see Chapter 11)
- Angiotensin II receptor antagonists (see Chapter 12).

Angiotensin II receptor antagonists are the newest group to be intro-duced and data on this group are necessarily more limited at the moment. Each class acts at different sites (see individual drug chapters), although the precise mechanism is not understood in all cases. The classes show major differences in adverse effects and ancillary properties that make them particularly suitable for patients with certain conditions and which also mean they are contraindicated in other patients. Management Focus (see p. 33) outlines these indications and contraindications, highlighting the differences between the main classes. Further details are given in the individual drug chapters.

There are various other antihypertensive drugs that are covered in the chapter on miscellaneous drugs (Chapter 13). Some of these have uses in special circumstances but many are associated with various adverse effects that limit their use.

Studies that have compared different classes of drugs

When comparing antihypertensive drugs in terms of blood pressure control, side-effects or quality of life, studies such as the TOMHS[1] (comparing chlortalidone, acebutolol, amlodipine, enalapril and doxazosin), a similar study[2] (comparing hydrochlorothiazide, atenolol, diltiazem, captopril, prazosin and clonidine) and HANE[3] (comparing hydrochlorothiazide, atenolol, nitrendipine and enalapril) have all shown that response to, and tolerance of, the six main types of antihypertensive drug is similar. Each type provides blood pressure control in about 50% of patients. The comparative studies did show, however, that there were differences in average response between drug classes related to age[4] and ethnic group.[5]

Studies of efficacy in reducing cardiovascular mortality

Ideally, there needs to be trial evidence that the drugs used to treat hypertension, as well as reducing blood pressure, also reduce cardiovascular mortality and morbidity. Such studies are often referred to as outcome trials. Most of the evidence from outcome trials is for thiazides and/or beta blockers since these have been the mainstays of hypertension management for longest. Overall these outcome trials have shown significant reductions in stroke (by 38%), in coronary events (by 16%), and in cardiovascular mortality (by 21%). The absolute benefit from treatment is smaller in women than men but this is compatible with their lower cardiovascular risk.

Evidence is emerging for reduced mortality and morbidity with calcium-channel blockers and ACE inhibitors. Studies of calcium-channel blockers in hypertensive patients have produced similar reductions in stroke risks to those found in studies involving thiazides or beta blockers.[6–8] However, these studies have recorded too few coronary heart

MANAGEMENT FOCUS

Drug choice

Drug	Indications*	Contraindications*
Thiazides	Elderly (isolated systolic hypertension)	Gout (dyslipidaemia)
Beta blockers	Post myocardial infarction, angina (tachyarrhythmias, heart failure†, essential tremor, hyperthyroidism, migraine)	Asthma/chronic obstructive pulmonary disease, heart block (heart failure†, dyslipidaemia, peripheral vascular disease, physically active patients)
ACE inhibitors	Left ventricular dysfunction, heart failure, type 1 diabetic nephropathy (type 2 diabetic nephropathy, post myocardial infarction)	Renovascular disease (peripheral vascular disease, renal impairment)
Calcium-channel blockers — Dihydropyridine type	Elderly with isolated systolic hypertension (angina)	
Calcium-channel blockers — Verapamil/diltiazem	Angina (myocardial infarction, atrial tachycardia and fibrillation)	Heart block, heart failure
Alpha blockers	Benign prostatic hyperplasia (dyslipidaemia, glucose intolerance)	Urinary incontinence (postural hypotension)
Angiotensin II receptor antagonists	ACE inhibitor-induced cough (heart failure)	Renovascular disease (peripheral vascular disease, renal impairment)

*Conditions appearing within brackets are regarded as being possible indications/contraindications.
†Beta blockers are contraindicated in uncontrolled heart failure, but may be used in certain cases of heart failure.

disease events for any conclusions to be drawn of the effect of calcium-channel blockers on this outcome. The CAPPP study[9] compared captopril with other antihypertensive therapy (mainly diuretic or beta blocker-based regimens) and found that the overall effect on cardiovascular morbidity and mortality was similar in the two groups. Captopril was associated with a lower total cardiovascular mortality, but fatal and non-fatal strokes were more common in patients receiving captopril, possibly because of a higher average diastolic blood pressure at entry to the study.

Until outcome trials are available for the other classes of anti-hypertensive drugs, evidence for their benefit rests on studies that show reductions in surrogate markers, such as left ventricular hypertrophy or microproteinuria. However, only outcome trials will demonstrate whether these markers correlate with effects on cardiovascular mortality and morbidity.

Persistent excess cardiovascular risk

An important issue uncovered by these outcome trials is that treated hypertensive patients still have a persistent excess risk of coronary and stroke death compared with normotensive subjects. There are many factors that could be contributing to this excess risk. It has been a concern that one of the factors may be that both thiazides and beta blockers cause metabolic disturbances, including dose-dependent changes in lipids and glucose tolerance. Beta blockers may also promote weight gain. It has been feared that these effects, which increase a patient's cardiovascular risk, could be offsetting the benefits of reducing blood pressure. However, the CAPPP study,[9] comparing an ACE inhibitor regimen with diuretics and beta blockers, found that outcome was similar in both groups. The study did find, though, that more patients assigned to beta blockers or thiazides (21% more) developed diabetes over 5 years when compared with treatment based on an ACE inhibitor, although another study[10] found that, while beta blockers increased the risk of developing diabetes over a 6-year period, patients taking thiazides showed no increased risk. It was hoped that a large comparative study (part of ALLHAT[11]) would show whether metabolically neutral classes of antihypertensive drugs would improve cardiovascular outcomes. The study compared doxazosin (an alpha blocker that has no effect on lipids or glucose metabolism) with the thiazide-related diuretic chlortalidone. The doxazosin arm of the trial was terminated early; interim analysis of the results found that, while doxazosin and chlortalidone had similar effects on risk of coronary heart disease death or non-fatal myocardial infarction, chlortalidone was associated with a significantly lower risk of combined cardio-vascular events (especially congestive heart failure).

Calcium-channel blockers

The role of calcium-channel blockers in hypertension has caused much controversy over recent years.[12] The controversy has arisen over reports associating dihydropyridine calcium-channel blockers with increased risk of coronary events, cancer, bleeding, depression, suicide and other adverse events.[12–14] However, these associations have come from observational or small randomised studies that are subject to bias and confounding. These concerns about safety have not been supported by evidence from controlled studies of dihydropyridine calcium-channel blockers such as PRAISE,[15] STONE[8] and Syst-Eur.[6] Results from two large comparative studies, ASCOT and ALLHAT, that are currently underway are awaited to clarify further the role of calcium-channel blockers. Short-acting formulations of nifedipine should no longer be used for hypertension since their use may be associated with large variations in blood pressure and tachycardia. The British Hypertension Society (BHS) guidelines[16] consider that, apart from this caveat, the available evidence suggests that the benefits of dihydropyridine calcium-channel blockers exceed any risks when they are prescribed for appropriate indications.

To summarise, the six major classes of antihypertensive drug are similar in terms of their effects on blood pressure and tolerability. However, since thiazides and beta blockers have the greatest body of evidence showing they reduce cardiovascular morbidity and mortality, these are the drugs of first choice in the straightforward patient with no contraindications to these agents. ACE inhibitors, alpha blockers, calcium-channel blockers and angiotensin II receptor antagonists are considered alternative first-choice drugs in patients with contraindications to thiazides and beta blockers.[16–18] They may also be first-choice drugs in patients who have concomitant conditions that are specific indications for these drugs (see Management Focus, p. 33).

Selecting the appropriate drug for the individual patient

As discussed above, there may be specific indications and contraindications that influence drug choice in a particular patient. Other factors that should be considered are listed in Management Focus (below). However, it should be remembered that for the individual patient, one drug may work well or poorly and susceptibility to adverse effects is unpredictable. Some patients respond better to one type of drug than another but no single factor explains why those who respond do so.

Principles of drug treatment

Regardless of which particular drug is chosen for a patient, there are a few principles that govern the use of antihypertensive drugs.

- Start with a low dose to minimise adverse effects. If there is a good blood pressure response and the drug is well tolerated, the dose can be increased gradually until the target blood pressure is reached (see below for initiation of treatment).
- Use drug combinations (see below) to maximise blood pressure response and minimise adverse effects.
- Change to a different drug class if initial doses of the first drug do not produce much effect on blood pressure or if side-effects are a problem.
- Use formulations that give at least 24-hour blood pressure control. This is important for compliance and also to ensure that blood pressure is controlled in the early morning when a surge in blood pressure occurs (with increased cardiovascular risk). Avoiding blood pressure variation throughout the day also helps avoid target organ damage.

MANAGEMENT FOCUS

Factors influencing choice of drug

- Any contraindications to drugs
- Presence of target organ damage, clinical cardiovascular disease, renal disease or diabetes
- Cardiovascular risk factor profile of the patient
- Coexisting disorders that either favour or limit the use of particular classes of antihypertensive drugs
- Interactions with drugs used for other conditions in the patient
- Age of patient
- Race
- Occupation of patient (e.g. driver)
- Lifestyle (e.g. sporting activities, sexual activity)

Initiating drug therapy

Having decided which drug to use, treatment is started at the lowest recommended dose and gradually titrated upwards until the blood pressure is reduced to the target pressure (see Chapter 3) or side-effects intervene. Thiazides are the exception to this, as the dose–response curve is very flat and the maximum effect on blood pressure is achieved at low doses. Increasing the dose further only increases the side-effects.

Most patients only need a very gradual reduction in blood pressure. The fall in blood pressure should be relatively small and gradual to allow for maintenance of blood flow to vital organs. An interval of at least 4 weeks should be allowed to observe the full response unless it is necessary to lower blood pressure more urgently.

The patient should be questioned about adverse effects that may be expected with whichever drug has been chosen. Patients may assume that some side-effects are inevitable and they may not realise that switching to another class of drug may remove the unwanted effect. Compliance with treatment should also be assessed.

In about half of all patients with hypertension, the first drug tried will fail to produce a sufficient response in blood pressure. If the drug is well tolerated and the hypertension is mild and uncomplicated, substitution of a drug from another class should be tried. Several classes of drug may need to be tried before a satisfactory treatment is found. If the drug is well tolerated but the hypertension is more severe or complicated, addition of a second (and third) drug (if necessary) is advised as the priority is to reduce blood pressure as quickly as possible. Treatment can be stepped down later if the blood pressure falls substantially below the optimal level.

See Management Focus (p. 27) for a summary of the stages of management of a patient with hypertension.

Drug combinations[19,20]

The majority of patients with hypertension will need combination drug therapy to control their blood pressure satisfactorily. The HOT study[21] found that one-third of the patients studied needed three or more drugs to achieve satisfactory blood pressure control; fewer than one-third were controlled by monotherapy. The UKPDS study[22] of hypertension in patients with type 2 diabetes reported similar findings.

The major classes of drug generally have additive effects on blood pressure when they are prescribed together. Thus, combination therapy allows lower doses of the individual drugs to be used, with a consequent reduction in adverse effects. The most effective combinations involve drugs that act on different physiological systems. Examples of rational two-drug combinations are given in Management Focus (see below). Suitable three-drug combinations are a diuretic, ACE inhibitor and calcium-channel blocker or a diuretic, beta blocker and calcium-channel blocker. Certain drug combinations should not be used, for example, a beta blocker with either verapamil or probably diltiazem, an ACE inhibitor with an angiotensin II receptor antagonist, or a potassium-sparing diuretic with an ACE inhibitor.

Fixed-dose combinations are not widely used in the UK as they tend to be expensive and the dose of the individual components is not always appropriate. However, they are convenient for patients and may improve compliance. Their use should be considered once a patient has been stabilised on the components of the combination taken separately.

MANAGEMENT FOCUS

Two-drug combinations		
Two-drug combinations		*Comments*
Thiazide diuretic	+ Beta blocker	Beta blocker can counteract diuretic-induced increases in renin activity
	+ ACE inhibitor	Useful in blacks – diuretic activates renin–angiotensin system, may also prevent potassium depletion
Beta blocker	+ Calcium-channel blocker (except verapamil and possibly diltiazem)	Beta blocker inhibits sympathetic response to dihydropyridine calcium-channel blockers
	+ Alpha blocker	
Calcium-channel blocker	+ ACE inhibitor	Combination with dihydropyridine calcium-channel blocker may reduce proteinuria more than either drug alone, also less pedal oedema
Alpha blocker	+ Any other antihypertensive drug	

Resistant patients

In some patients, blood pressure remains above the target level despite trials of several different classes and combinations of drugs in adequate doses and institution of lifestyle measures. Such hypertension may be termed refractory hypertension. There are various factors that can contribute to resistant hypertension[23,24] (see Risk Factor Focus, below) and these patients require further investigation to discover the cause of their resistance and probably referral to a specialist.

Large doses of a loop diuretic can help to bring resistant hypertension under control in some patients. The combination of an ACE inhibitor and a calcium-channel blocker may also be effective in severe and resistant cases.

RISK FACTOR FOCUS

Factors contributing to resistant hypertension

- Non-compliance
- Inadequate drug dosage
- Inappropriate drug combination
- Drug interactions (see Risk Factor Focus, p. 9, for drugs causing hypertension)
- Excessive salt intake impairs the antihypertensive effect of some antihypertensives
- Salt sensitivity, especially in elderly and black patients (salt restriction may improve blood pressure control)
- Renal impairment – thiazides are often ineffective
- Unidentified secondary causes of hypertension (see Risk Factor Focus, p. 9)
- Associated conditions
  - Smoking
  - Increasing obesity
  - Insulin resistance
  - Excessive alcohol intake
  - Anxiety-induced hyperventilation/panic attacks
  - Chronic pain
- Pseudoresistance
  - 'White coat' hypertension
  - Pseudohypertension in older patients (false high blood pressure readings because of rigidity of arteries)
  - Use of too small a cuff on obese arm (produces high blood pressure readings)

References

1. Neaton J D, Grimm R H, Prineas R J, *et al*. Treatment of mild hypertension study: final results. *JAMA* 1993; 270: 713–724.
2. Materson B J, Reda D J, Cushman W C, *et al*. Single-drug therapy for hypertension in men: a comparison of six antihypertensive agents with placebo. *N Engl J Med* 1993; 328: 914–921. Correction *ibid*. 1994; 330: 1689.
3. Philipp T, Anlauf M, Distler A, *et al*. Randomised, double blind, multicentre comparison of hydrochlorothiazide, atenolol, nitrendipine, and enalapril in antihypertensive treatment: results of the HANE study. *BMJ* 1997; 315: 154–159.
4. Bennett N E. Hypertension in the elderly. *Lancet* 1994; 344: 447–449.
5. Kaplan N M. Ethnic aspects of hypertension. *Lancet* 1994; 344: 450–452.
6. Forette F, Seux M L, Staessen J A, *et al*. Prevention of dementia in randomised placebo controlled systolic hypertension in Europe (Syst-Eur) trial. *Lancet* 1998; 352: 1347–1351.
7. Liu L, Wang J G, Gong L, *et al*. Comparison of active treatment and placebo in older Chinese patients with isolated systolic hypertension. Systolic Hypertension in China (Syst-China) Collaborative Group. *J Hypertens* 1998; 16: 1823–1829.
8. Gong L, Zhang W, Zhu Y, *et al*. Shanghai trial of nifedipine in the elderly (STONE). *J Hypertens* 1996; 14: 1237–1245.
9. Hansson L, Lindholm L H, Niskanen L, *et al*. Effect of angiotensin-converting enzyme inhibition compared with conventional therapy on cardiovascular morbidity and mortality in hypertension: the Captopril Prevention Project (CAPPP). *Lancet* 1999; 353: 611–616.
10. Gress T W, Nieto F J, Shahar E, *et al*. Hypertension and antihypertensive therapy as risk factors for type 2 diabetes. *N Engl J Med* 2000; 342: 909–912.
11. ALLHAT Collaborative Research Group. Major cardiovascular events in hypertensive patients randomized to doxazosin vs chlorthalidone: the antihypertensive and lipid-lowering treatment to prevent heart attack trial (ALLHAT). *JAMA* 2000; 283: 1967–1975.
12. Cutler J A. Calcium-channel blockers for hypertension – uncertainty continues. *N Engl J Med* 1998; 338: 679–681.
13. Stanton AV. Calcium channel blockers. *BMJ* 1998; 316: 1471–1473.
14. Ad Hoc Subcommittee of the Liaison Committee of the World Health Organization and the International Society of Hypertension. Effects of calcium antagonists on the risks of coronary heart disease, cancer and bleeding. *J Hypertens* 1997; 15: 105–115.
15. O'Connor C M, Carson P E, Miller A B, *et al*. Effect of amlodipine on mode of death among patients with advanced heart failure in the PRAISE trial. Prospective Randomized Amlodipine Survival Evaluation. *Am J Cardiol* 1998; 82: 881–887.
16. Ramsay L E, Williams B, Johnston G D, *et al*. BHS guidelines. Guidelines for management of hypertension: report of the third working party of the British Hypertension Society. *J Hum Hypertens* 1999; 13: 569–592.
17. Joint National Committee. The sixth report of the Joint National Committee on prevention, detection, evaluation, and treatment of high blood pressure

(JNC VI). *Arch Intern Med* 1997; 157: 2413–2446. Correction *ibid.* 1998; 158: 573.

18. Guidelines Subcommittee. 1999 World Health Organization–International Society of Hypertension guidelines for the management of hypertension. *J Hypertens* 1999; 17: 151–183.

19. Opie L H, Messerli F H, eds. *Combination Drug Therapy for Hypertension.* New York: Lippincott-Raven, 1997.

20. Lip G Y, Beevers M, Beevers D G. The 'Birmingham hypertension square' for the optimum choice of add-in drugs for the management of resistant hypertension. *J Hum Hypertens* 1998; 12: 761–763.

21. Hansson L, Zanchetti A, Carruthers S G, *et al.* Effects of intensive blood-pressure lowering and low-dose aspirin in patients with hypertension: principal results of the Hypertension Optimal Treatment (HOT) randomised trial. *Lancet* 1998; 351: 1755–1762.

22. UK Prospective Diabetes Study Group. Tight blood pressure control and risk of macrovascular and microvascular complications in type 2 diabetes: UKPDS 38. *BMJ* 1998; 317: 703–713.

23. McInnes G T, Semple P F. Hypertension: investigation, assessment and diagnosis. *Br Med Bull* 1994; 50: 443–459.

24. Padfield P L. Resistant hypertension. *Prescribers' J* 1997; 37: 69–76.

5

Hypertension management in special patient groups

Some patients with hypertension have co-morbid conditions, such as renal disease or heart failure, which may influence the choice of anti-hypertensive agent or alter management in some way. Certain groups of patients, such as children or pregnant women, may also require different management. This chapter discusses the management of hypertension in the elderly patient, in patients with diabetes and in patients from ethnic minorities. For further information on the management of hypertension in other special patient groups, see the recommended reading list towards the end of the book.

Older patients[1,2]

In most westernised countries blood pressure rises with age. Thus, the prevalence of hypertension in the elderly (patients over the age of 60) is very high. Two patterns of hypertension are seen in the elderly: combined systolic and diastolic hypertension and isolated systolic hypertension. Isolated systolic hypertension is described and defined on p. 8. By age 80 years, a third of the population has isolated systolic hypertension. Isolated systolic hypertension is associated with significantly increased risk of cardiovascular mortality.

The elderly have tended to be undertreated in the past because the rise in blood pressure with age was widely regarded as inevitable. It was also considered that isolated systolic hypertension was not linked to increased cardiovascular mortality. In addition, there may have been a reluctance to treat adequately because of concerns that the elderly might tolerate antihypertensive therapy poorly. These concerns have not been upheld by analysis of adverse effects of outcome trials.[3]

Since age is one of the risk factors for cardiovascular events, elderly patients have a higher risk of cardiovascular complications than do younger people with the same blood pressures. This higher cardiovascular risk means that elderly hypertensives derive a greater benefit from antihypertensive treatment. Outcome trials have shown clear benefit from lowering blood pressure in elderly people up to the age of 80 years.[4-7] Heart failure and dementia are important consequences of hypertension in elderly patients and drug treatment of hypertension in this age group has been reported to reduce the incidence of heart failure by 50%;[8] dementia may also be reduced by antihypertensive treatment.[9] One ongoing trial, the Hypertension in the Very Elderly Trial, will provide data on treating hypertension in patients aged over 80 years.

Lifestyle measures are as effective as in younger patients and should continue to be promoted in the elderly. Antihypertensive therapy is indicated and clearly beneficial in people aged 60 years or more when systolic blood pressure is >160 mmHg, even if diastolic blood pressure is within normal limits.

Antihypertensive treatment of elderly patients with borderline isolated systolic hypertension (140–159/<90 mmHg) is advised when there are cardiovascular complications or evidence of target organ damage. There are no clear recommendations for management of elderly people with borderline isolated systolic hypertension who do not have these complications. Most of these patients will have an estimated 10-year coronary heart disease risk in excess of 15% simply because of their age and, on this basis, would be expected to benefit from antihypertensive therapy. However, the high prevalence of borderline isolated systolic hypertension in the elderly means that drug treatment would be needed for vast numbers of people, with enormous cost implications. The British Hypertension Society (BHS)[10] therefore recommends that a decision to treat with drugs should be made on an individual basis, taking into account the patient's general health and the anticipated benefit of treatment.

The management of very elderly patients with hypertension (those over the age of 80 years) will depend on the general level of health and concomitant disease. Elderly patients who were started on antihypertensive treatment before the age of 80 should continue their treatment beyond 80 years of age. When hypertension is first diagnosed after age 80, antihypertensive therapy should be considered if they are generally fit and have reasonable life expectancy, particularly if they have hypertensive complications or target organ damage.

Older patients tolerate antihypertensive treatment as well as younger age groups, although certain precautions need to be considered (see below). A low dose of a thiazide is the clear drug of first choice and is safe and effective in the elderly. Meta-analyses suggest that beta blockers decrease stroke but no other cardiovascular events in this age group.[11] The Syst-Eur study[7] showed that a dihydropyridine calcium-channel blocker is a suitable alternative for elderly hypertensives when thiazides are ineffective, contraindicated or not tolerated.

For patients with isolated systolic hypertension, there is now good trial evidence for the use of a low-dose thiazide or a long-acting dihydropyridine calcium-channel blocker as the first-line drug. BHS guidelines[10] recommend that target blood pressure levels on treatment should be similar to those of younger patients if possible.

Blood pressure measurement in the elderly

There are certain considerations that need to be borne in mind when measuring blood pressure in elderly patients. The 'white coat' effect is more common in the elderly. The elderly are also more likely to show pseudohypertension due to the stiffness of the large arteries, producing false high readings. Blood pressure should be measured in both the sitting and standing positions to see if there is orthostatic hypotension.

Cautions necessary to observe in the elderly

Antihypertensive therapy can be well tolerated in elderly patients, although there are various characteristics of the ageing process that mean it is more important in this age group that therapy is initiated slowly and gradually. Some of the factors that need to be borne in mind when using antihypertensives (and any drugs in the elderly) are listed in Risk Factor Focus (see p. 46).

Patients from ethnic minorities

Hypertension is common amongst blacks, with prevalence as high as 50% in those over the age of 40 years. Black hypertensives seem particularly prone to complications, notably stroke, renal failure and left ventricular hypertrophy. The first-choice antihypertensive drug in the straightforward patient is a thiazide diuretic. Beta blockers may be less effective in blacks as black people tend to have lower renin levels than whites. Angiotensin-converting enzyme (ACE) inhibitors and angiotensin II receptor antagonists therefore also tend to be less effective. However, these drugs should not be withheld in patients who have specific indications for them. Relative resistance can be overcome by using high doses, by adding a diuretic or by reducing salt

RISK FACTOR FOCUS

Factors that might contribute to increased risk of antihypertensive treatment in the elderly

Factors	Potential complications
Impaired baroreceptor sensitivity	Orthostatic hypotension
Impaired cerebral autoregulation	Cerebral ischaemia with small falls in systemic pressure
Reduced intravascular volume	Orthostatic hypotension Volume depletion Hyponatraemia
Sensitivity to hypokalaemia	Arrhythmia Muscle weakness
Reduced renal function	Drug accumulation. Susceptibility to renal impairment with ACE inhibitors
Reduced hepatic function	Drug accumulation
Polypharmacy	Drug interactions
Central nervous system changes	Depression Confusion – contributes to poor compliance
Increased prevalence of heart failure	Reduced tolerance of agents with negative inotropic action

intake. Response to ACE inhibitors can also be improved by combination with calcium-channel blockers or alpha blockers. Restriction of salt intake is often necessary to achieve good blood pressure control in blacks. In some hypertensives without evidence of target organ damage, a low-salt diet may sometimes obviate the need for antihypertensive drugs.

British South Asians (from the Indian subcontinent) also have a high prevalence of hypertension. Insulin resistance and type 2 diabetes are also particularly common. They are at increased risk of stroke and particularly high risk of coronary heart disease. Management of hypertension therefore requires particular emphasis on control of glucose levels and lipid levels in addition to adequate control of blood pressure. Response to the different antihypertensive drug classes seems to be the same as in white Europeans, although evidence is limited. Concomitant aspirin or statin therapy should be considered given the high risk of coronary heart disease in this group.

Hypertension in diabetes

Patients with diabetes and hypertension are at very high risk of both cardiovascular complications and microvascular disease (diabetic nephropathy and retinopathy). Hypertension is common in diabetes. The prevalence differs in type 1 and 2 diabetes. In type 1 diabetes, in the absence of nephropathy, the prevalence of hypertension is similar to that in the non-diabetic population. Hypertension is common in type 2 diabetes and in type 1 diabetes with nephropathy.

The lifestyle measures recommended for patients with hypertension are similar to those recommended for patients with diabetes anyway and are important for controlling cardiovascular risk. Strict glycaemic control is also important. The high risk of cardiovascular complications in patients with both diabetes and hypertension necessitates the initiation of drug therapy when blood pressure is ≥140/90 mmHg.

The choice of antihypertensive drug depends on the presence of nephropathy. ACE inhibitors seem to have a specific renoprotective effect in type 1 diabetes and nephropathy.[12] They also delay progression from microalbuminuria to overt nephropathy[13] and reduce progression of retinopathy. The dose of ACE inhibitor should be titrated to the maximum recommended and tolerated. Strict blood pressure control is important to prevent renal deterioration and a recommended target blood pressure is <130/80 mmHg, with an even lower target blood pressure (<125/75 mmHg) where proteinuria exceeds 1 g in 24 hours.[10] These blood pressure targets will probably necessitate the use of other antihypertensive drugs in addition to an ACE inhibitor. An alpha blocker, calcium-channel blocker, thiazide or cardioselective beta blocker are all suitable additional agents. Patients who fail to tolerate an ACE inhibitor because of persistent cough may be switched to an angiotensin II receptor antagonist, although the results of trials are awaited to confirm a renoprotective effect with this class of drug.

The role of ACE inhibitors in patients with type 2 diabetes and nephropathy is less clear. As in type 1 diabetes, they may slow progression from microalbuminuria to overt nephropathy, but it is not certain whether they have a specific renoprotective effect in type 2 diabetes with nephropathy. Blood pressure reduction itself slows the progression of nephropathy in these patients and any benefits seen with ACE inhibitors may be due solely to their antihypertensive action.

The optimal antihypertensive drug for patients with type 1 or type 2 diabetes and no evidence of nephropathy or microalbuminuria has yet to be established. All the first-line antihypertensive drugs can be used.

There have been concerns over the use of beta blockers and thiazides because of their potential adverse effects on glucose and lipid metabolism; however, subgroup analyses of outcome trials have shown that both these groups of drugs are safe and effective in patients with diabetes. The recommended blood pressure target is <140/80 mmHg.[10]

Since patients with hypertension and diabetes are at high risk of cardiovascular complications, it is important that they should be considered for treatment with aspirin and/or a statin.

References

1. Kinirons M, Jackson S. Hypertension in the elderly. *Practitioner* 1997; 241: 686–690.
2. Bennet N E. Hypertension in the elderly. *Lancet* 1994; 344: 447–449.
3. Lever A F, Ramsay L E. Treatment of hypertension in the elderly. *J Hypertens* 1995; 13: 571–579.
4. Dahlöf B, Lindholm L H, Hansson L, *et al*. Morbidity and mortality in the Swedish Trial in Old Patients with Hypertension (STOP-Hypertension). *Lancet* 1991; 338: 1281–1285.
5. SHEP Cooperative Research Group. Prevention of stroke by antihypertensive drug treatment in older persons with isolated systolic hypertension: final results of the Systolic Hypertension in the Elderly Program (SHEP). *JAMA* 1991; 265: 3255–3264.
6. MRC Working Party. Medical Research Council trial of treatment of hypertension in older patients: principal results. *BMJ* 1992; 304: 405–412.
7. Staessen J A, Fagard R, Thijs L, *et al*. Randomised double-blind comparison of placebo and active treatment for older patients with isolated systolic hypertension. *Lancet* 1997; 350: 757–764. Correction *ibid*.: 1636.
8. Kostis J B, Davis B R, Culter J, *et al*. Prevention of heart failure by antihypertensive drug treatment in older persons with isolated systolic hypertension. SHEP Cooperative Research Group. *JAMA* 1997; 278: 212–216.
9. Forette F, Seux M L, Staessen J A, *et al*. Prevention of dementia in randomised double-blind placebo-controlled systolic hypertension in Europe (Syst-Eur) trial. *Lancet* 1998; 352: 1347–1351.
10. Ramsay L E, Williams B, Johnston G D, *et al*. BHS guidelines. Guidelines for management of hypertension: report of the third working party of the British Hypertension Society. *J Hum Hypertens* 1999; 13: 569–592.
11. Messerli F H, Grossman E, Goldbourt U. Are β-blockers efficacious as first-line therapy for hypertension in the elderly? A systematic review. *JAMA* 1998; 279: 1903–1907.
12. Lewis E J, Hunsicker L G, Bain R P, Rohde R D. The effect of angiotensin-converting-enzyme inhibition on diabetic nephropathy. *N Engl J Med* 1993; 329: 1456–1462.
13. Cooper M E. Pathogenesis, prevention, and treatment of diabetic nephropathy. *Lancet* 1998; 352: 213–219.

6

Lifestyle management

Lifestyle management (sometimes referred to as non-pharmacological management or hygienic measures) involves modifying various lifestyle habits with the aim of reducing blood pressure and also reducing overall cardiovascular risk. It is promoted both for individual patients with hypertension and for whole populations as part of a primary prevention strategy.

Individual patients

As trials of drug treatment have demonstrated benefit for patients with even mild hypertension, so the population of patients who are candidates for antihypertensive drug therapy has grown. This has considerable economic costs and personal costs of lifelong medication. Changes in diet and lifestyle have been shown to lower blood pressure and may also reduce associated cardiovascular risk factors.[1-4] More emphasis has therefore been placed on lifestyle measures which can be used as sole therapy in patients with mild hypertension and, when used in conjunction with antihypertensive drugs, can reduce the dose and/or the number of drugs needed. Conversely, the response to antihypertensive drugs is reduced in patients who fail to make the necessary changes in lifestyle. The lifestyle modifications that are recommended in guidelines are listed in Management Focus (see p. 50). Some other measures that have also been promoted but have less evidence of benefit are listed at the end of the chapter (see p. 54). In patients with mild hypertension, but no cardiovascular complications or target organ damage, the response to these measures should be observed during the initial 4–6-month period of evaluation. When drug therapy has to be introduced more quickly, for example in patients with severe hypertension, non-pharmacological measures should be instituted in parallel with drug treatment.

Primary prevention

An even greater possible value for lifestyle measures is their potential for reducing blood pressure even a small amount in the broader community.

MANAGEMENT FOCUS

Principal lifestyle measures
• Reduce weight (if overweight) • Reduce alcohol intake • Reduce salt intake • Increase physical exercise • Stop smoking • Increase fruit and vegetable consumption • Reduce fat intake

This would have the effect of delaying, if not preventing, the development of hypertension and thereby having a much greater impact on the overall level of cardiovascular disease in a population than the individual approach of treating only those with established disease. It is estimated that a reduction of just 2–3 mmHg in the population blood pressure would produce the same benefits as drug treatment of all hypertensive patients with a diastolic blood pressure greater than 105 mmHg. In addition to the beneficial effect on blood pressure, promotion of lifestyle measures in the whole population would also reduce other cardiovascular risk factors. The lifestyle changes recommended for patients with hypertension are therefore promoted for the entire population. (See Chapter 15 for further information on primary prevention.)

Compliance

It is important to note that changes in lifestyle may be difficult to achieve and it may be unrealistic to expect people to adopt several measures all at once; the objective should therefore be to achieve these changes over a period of months. The aim should be to produce permanent changes in lifestyle. Although many patients do not adhere to lifestyle measures, the same is true of drug therapy. The same techniques that are used to improve patient compliance with drug therapy (see Chapter 16) should be used to ensure that lifestyle measures are also adhered to.

Counselling is an important aspect of ensuring compliance with lifestyle measures. The TONE study[4] of non-pharmacological interventions in elderly patients found that structured counselling about losing weight and reducing sodium intake safely reduced the need for antihypertensive treatment in the elderly. Well-written clear information also helps improve compliance.

Principal lifestyle measures

The main lifestyle measures that should be adopted are listed in Management Focus (see p. 50) and outlined in more detail below. There have been various other measures (see p. 54) that have been advocated by some, although the evidence for benefit is doubtful.

Weight loss

The Intersalt study of 52 communities worldwide found that weight among all the characteristics measured (except age) had the strongest and most consistent correlation with blood pressure.[5] Many patients with hypertension are overweight and therefore weight reduction by calorie restriction is appropriate in these patients; for those who are obese, weight reduction should be regarded as a major priority. Weight loss may result in a blood pressure reduction of about 2.5/1.5 mmHg for each kg lost.[1,4] It should also be borne in mind that calorie restriction may improve other coronary risk factors in the hypertensive patient, such as dyslipidaemia and insulin resistance.

Various mechanisms have been suggested whereby increasing weight increases blood pressure and vice versa. Activity of the sympathetic nervous system is considered the most likely mechanism.

Compliance with weight-reducing diets poses a significant problem and many patients will not maintain a weight reduction diet long-term. Dietary changes should be introduced gradually to aid compliance. It may be useful to question patients on their current eating habits and then select areas for change. Referral to a dietician may be helpful in some cases. The aim should be for less than 33% of the total calorie intake to be made up of fat, with less than one-third of this being saturated fat. This may be achieved particularly by limiting the amount of animal fat consumed (dairy products, fatty meat).

Reduce alcohol intake

Alcohol intake above 21 units per week is associated with a rise in blood pressure that is reversible when intake is reduced.[6] The effect is a chronic one and the response to alcohol reduction emerges slowly, peaking at about 4–6 weeks. Binge drinking is also associated with an increased risk of stroke.[7] The mechanism for a reduction in blood pressure with alcohol restriction is unknown; reduced sympathetic nervous system activity seems likely. Patients should be advised to moderate alcohol consumption to the current recommended limit of no more than 21 units a week for men and 14 for women (1 unit = $\frac{1}{2}$ pint beer/lager = 1 glass of wine = 1 'short' measure of spirits). Reducing alcohol intake will also assist weight loss. Consumption of smaller amounts of alcohol, up to the recommended limit, may protect against coronary heart disease[8] and should not be discouraged. A reduction in alcohol intake is associated with a potentially disadvantageous fall in high-density lipoprotein (HDL)-cholesterol but this is prevented by simultaneous calorie restriction.

Reduce salt intake

The role of salt restriction in hypertension has caused much controversy over the years. Nevertheless, it is generally agreed that reducing the amount of salt consumed in the diet is beneficial. Salt reduction from an average of 10 to 5 g (5 g = 1 teaspoon) daily has been reported to lower blood pressure by about 5/3 mmHg,[4,9,10] with larger blood pressure falls in the elderly and those with higher initial blood pressure levels.[10] Blacks also generally show a larger response to salt restriction.

A high salt intake can impair the efficacy of some antihypertensive drugs. Therefore moderate salt restriction may not only reduce blood pressure but can also potentiate the antihypertensive action of these drugs. This is particularly marked in the case of angiotensin-converting enzyme (ACE) inhibitors, but it has also been demonstrated with diuretics and with beta blockers. Patients on calcium-channel blockers show no effect of salt restriction. Moderate salt restriction will also reduce the potassium loss induced by diuretics.

Most people eat around 10 g of salt a day. The British Hypertension Society (BHS) guidelines[11] recommend that patients should be advised to reduce this to 5 g daily (or 2 g sodium daily). The elderly, in particular, tend to use a lot of salt since many lose some of the perception of saltiness. Patients should be advised to avoid adding salt to cooking or at the table (taste preference for salt diminishes after a few months on a lower-salt diet). However, this alone will not produce a sufficiently large reduction in salt consumption and patients need to avoid other sources of salt in their diet. For example, canned, processed or precooked foods tend to contain large amounts of salt, as do flavour enhancers such as stock cubes or bottled sauces. Other foods high in salt include some breakfast cereals, bread, most cheese, savoury snacks, bacon and ham. Sodium is also present in large amounts in some antacids and some beverages. Generally, if the sodium content is more than 0.2 g/100 g of food, the food is high in salt and these foods should be avoided.

Most fresh foods contain little salt and consumption of these should be recommended. The effect of salt restriction seems to be enhanced by consumption of foods rich in potassium (e.g. fresh fruit and vegetables).[12]

Some patients use salt substitutes containing potassium chloride; while these may be beneficial, there is the risk of hyperkalaemia when these salt substitutes are combined with ACE inhibitors or potassium-sparing diuretics. Some patients may use rock salt or sea salt with the perception that these are 'healthy' alternatives to table salt, but this is not the case.

Physical exercise

Although acute exercise increases blood pressure by an amount that depends on the degree of fitness and level of exertion, regular exercise, such as taking 30–45 minutes of modest aerobic exercise (a brisk walk or a swim) three times a week actually produces a modest fall in blood pressure. The mechanism of this effect is not known; reduced sympathetic nervous system activity may be responsible. Increasing exercise also contributes to weight loss.

Regular dynamic exercise, for example a brisk walk, is the type of exercise that is beneficial rather than isometric exercise, such as weight training. Exercise obviously needs to be tailored to the individual patient; for example, three vigorous training sessions a week may be appropriate for fit younger patients while brisk walking for 20 minutes a day is more suitable for older patients. The regular exercise needs to be maintained since the post-exercise reduction in blood pressure disappears about 2 weeks after the activity has stopped.[13]

Patients should be warned that beta blockers will curtail their exercise capacity (unlike other antihypertensives).

Smoking cessation

The most effective lifestyle measure to reduce overall cardiovascular risk is smoking cessation. Although stopping smoking has no effect on blood pressure, smoking multiplies the cardiovascular risk as much as two- to fivefold. Smoking was one factor related to the persistent excess coronary mortality in men with treated hypertension.[14] Cardiovascular mortality and morbidity fall within a few months of stopping smoking.[15] In particular there are large reductions in risk among those who quit before 35 years of age or middle age; life expectancy in these patients is typically equal to that of lifelong non-smokers.

It is important, then, that hypertensive patients who smoke should be given advice and help to stop smoking.[16,17] Regular counselling has been shown to be the most effective way to help patients give up smoking. Nicotine replacement therapies (chewing gum, patches, inhalation, sublingual tablets or spray) approximately double smoking cessation rates[18] and should be used in conjunction with counselling where appropriate. It should be remembered that nicotine replacement products are contraindicated in patients with severe cardiovascular disease or recent stroke (including transient ischaemic attack) and should be used with caution in less severe cardiovascular disease or peripheral vascular disease. See *British National Formulary* Section 4.10 for more details on precautions and side-effects of nicotine replacement therapy.[19]

Increased fruit and vegetable consumption

Increasing daily consumption of fruit and vegetables from two to seven portions has been shown to lower blood pressure by about 7/3 mmHg in patients with hypertension.[1] Larger falls in blood pressure may be produced if a reduced-fat diet is also followed.[1] The effect of increased fruit and vegetable intake on blood pressure may be a consequence of increased potassium intake.[20,21]

Reduced total fat and saturated fat intake

Serum cholesterol level before and during the treatment of hypertension is an important predictor of cardiovascular disease.[14] All patients should be advised to reduce saturated fat and cholesterol intake, and to substitute polyunsaturated and monounsaturated fats. These dietary changes will reduce serum cholesterol by an average of 6%.[22] Compliance with a reduced-fat diet is often a problem and many patients do not maintain the dietary changes.[23] Many hypertensive patients need statin treatment in addition to dietary fat restriction (see p. 24). Increased consumption of oily fish is also recommended (see below).

Other measures

Other interventions tried, but with less evidence of benefit, include increased intake of calcium and magnesium, and relaxation therapies for stress reduction. Relaxation exercises and meditation lower blood pressure slightly but there is no convincing evidence of long-term benefit.

Calcium intake

Low dietary calcium intake is associated with an increased prevalence of hypertension and an increased calcium intake may lower blood pressure in some patients with hypertension. However, the overall effect is minimal and, while it is important to maintain calcium intake for general health, there is no rationale for recommending calcium supplements to lower blood pressure.

Magnesium intake

Although there is evidence to suggest that there may be an association between low dietary magnesium intake and higher blood pressure, there are no convincing data to justify recommending increased magnesium intake to reduce blood pressure.

Omega-3 fatty acids[24]

Large doses of fish oil may reduce blood pressure[25] but the large doses required can produce abdominal discomfort. However, although fish oils cannot be recommended for their blood pressure lowering effects, they are beneficial in reducing cardiovascular risk. The DOH has recommended consumption of two portions of fish a week, one of which should be oily.

References

1. Appel L J, Moore T J, Obarzanek E, *et al.* A clinical trial of the effects of dietary patterns on blood pressure. *N Engl J Med* 1997; 336: 1117–1124.
2. Applegate W B, Miller S T, Elam J T, *et al.* Nonpharmacologic intervention to reduce blood pressure in older patients with mild hypertension. *Arch Intern Med* 1992; 152: 1162–1166.
3. The Trials of Hypertension Prevention Collaborative Research Group. Effects of weight loss and sodium reduction intervention on blood pressure and hypertension incidence in overweight people with high-normal blood pressure. The Trials of Hypertension Prevention, phase II. *Arch Intern Med* 1997; 157: 657–667.
4. Whelton P K, Appel L J, Espeland M A, *et al.* Sodium reduction and weight loss in the treatment of hypertension in older persons: a randomized controlled trial of nonpharmacologic interventions in the elderly (TONE). *JAMA* 1998; 279: 839–846.
5. Intersalt Cooperative Research Group. Intersalt: an international study of electrolyte excretion and blood pressure: results for 24 hour urinary sodium and potassium excretion. *BMJ* 1988; 297: 319–328.
6. Kaplan N M. Alcohol and hypertension. *Lancet* 1995; 345: 1588–1589.

7. Gill J S, Zezulka A V, Shipley M J, *et al*. Stroke and alcohol consumption. *N Engl J Med* 1986; 315: 1041–1046.

8. McElduff P, Dobson A. How much alcohol and how often? Population based case-control study of alcohol consumption and risk of a major coronary event. *BMJ* 1997; 314: 1159–1164.

9. Law M R, Frost C D, Wald N J. By how much does dietary salt reduction lower blood pressure? III – Analysis of data from trials of salt reduction. *BMJ* 1991; 302: 819–824.

10. Midgley J P, Matthew A G, Greenwood C M T, Logan A G. Effect of reduced dietary sodium on blood pressure. A meta-analysis of randomized controlled trials. *JAMA* 1996; 275: 1590–1597.

11. Ramsay L E, Williams B, Johnston G D, *et al*. BHS guidelines. Guidelines for management of hypertension: report of the third working party of the British Hypertension Society. *J Hum Hypertens* 1999; 13: 569–592.

12. Sacks F M, Svetkey L P, Vollmer W M, *et al*. Effects on blood pressure of reduced dietary sodium and the Dietary Approaches to Stop Hypertension (DASH) diet. *N Engl J Med* 2001; 344: 3–10.

13. Arroll B, Beaglehole R. Exercise for hypertension. *Lancet* 1993: 341; 1248–1249.

14. Andersson O K, Almgren T, Persson B, *et al*. Survival in treated hypertension: follow up study after two decades. *BMJ* 1998; 317: 167–171.

15. Eagles C J, Martin U. Non-pharmacological modification of cardiac risk factors: part 3–smoking cessation and alcohol consumption. *J Clin Pharm Ther* 1998; 23: 1–9.

16. Snell M, ed. *Medicines Ethics and Practice 24: A Guide for Pharmacists*. London: RPSGB, July 2000.

17. West R, McNeill A, Raw M. Smoking cessation guidelines for health professionals: an update. *Thorax* 2000; 55: 987–999.

18. Raw M, McNeill A, West R. Smoking cessation: evidence based recommendations for the healthcare system. *BMJ* 1999; 318: 182–185.

19. Mehta D K, ed. *British National Formulary*, no. 40. London: British Medical Association/RPSGB, 2000.

20. Fortherby M D, Potter J F. Potassium supplementation reduces clinic and ambulatory blood pressure in elderly hypertensive patients. *J Hypertens* 1992; 10: 1403–1408.

21. Whelton P K, He J, Cutler J A, *et al*. Effects of oral potassium on blood pressure: meta-analysis of randomized controlled clinical trials. *JAMA* 1997; 277: 1624–1632.

22. Tang J L, Armitage J M, Lancaster T, *et al*. Systematic review of dietary intervention trials to lower blood total cholesterol in free-living subjects. *BMJ* 1998; 316: 1213–1220.

23. Imperial Cancer Research Fund OXCHECK Study Group. Effectiveness of health checks conducted by nurses in primary care: final results of the OXCHECK study. *BMJ* 1995; 310: 1099–1104.

24. Mason P. Fish oils – an update. *Pharm J* 2000; 265: 720–724.

25. Morris M C, Sacks F, Rosner B. Does fish oil lower blood pressure? A meta-analysis of controlled trials. *Circulation* 1993; 88: 523–533.

7

Thiazide and related diuretics

Indications

Thiazide diuretics are first-choice agents in hypertension. They may be used alone or can be combined with any of the other major antihypertensives; combination with an angiotensin-converting enzyme (ACE) inhibitor or a beta blocker is common. In some patient groups, such as blacks and the elderly, the thiazides are particularly efficacious.

Mechanism of action

Thiazide diuretics (also known as benzothiadiazides) were introduced into clinical practice in 1958. They were developed as a result of efforts to improve the metabolic and diuretic properties of carbonic anhydrase inhibitors. The first of the thiazides to be developed was chlorothiazide, a much less potent carbonic anhydrase inhibitor and much less prone to induce significant metabolic acidosis. Thiazide diuretics are all structurally similar in that they all contain a benzothiadiazine heterocycle (see Figure 7.1). There are various other diuretics that are related structurally to thiazides, although they lack the benzothiadiazine heterocycle, such as chlortalidone, indapamide, metolazone and xipamide. These related diuretics share the actions and effects of thiazides. Thiazide and related compounds were originally indicated for the treatment of disorders such as sodium and water retention secondary to heart failure and renal insufficiency; hypertension has actually turned out to be their major use.

Thiazide diuretics are moderately potent diuretics that exert their diuretic effect by inhibiting the transport of sodium and chloride across the epithelium from the tubular lumen in the early part of the distal convoluted tubule (cortical diluting segment) of the kidney. This results in the delivery of increased amounts of sodium to the distal tubule, where some of it is exchanged for potassium. The mechanism of action at the molecular level is still poorly understood.

Thiazide diuretics therefore increase the excretion of sodium and potassium ions, and consequently of water. The excretion of other

Thiazide diuretics

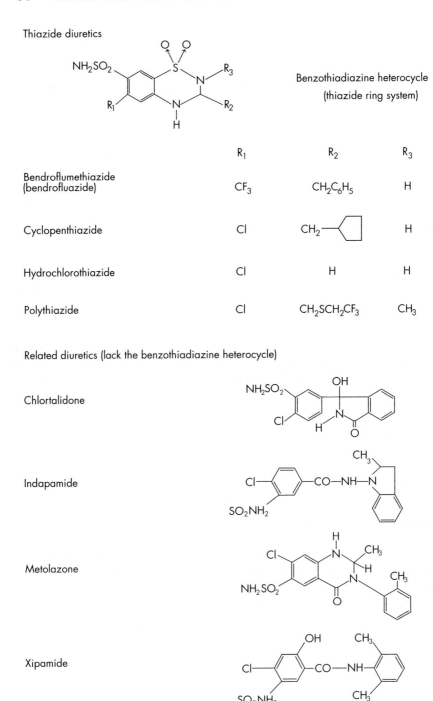

Benzothiadiazine heterocycle
(thiazide ring system)

	R_1	R_2	R_3
Bendroflumethiazide (bendrofluazide)	CF_3	$CH_2C_6H_5$	H
Cyclopenthiazide	Cl	CH₂—⬠	H
Hydrochlorothiazide	Cl	H	H
Polythiazide	Cl	$CH_2SCH_2CF_3$	CH_3

Related diuretics (lack the benzothiadiazine heterocycle)

Chlortalidone

Indapamide

Metolazone

Xipamide

Figure 7.1 Thiazide and related diuretics.

electrolytes, notably magnesium, is also increased. The excretion of calcium is reduced. Thiazide diuretics also reduce carbonic anhydrase activity so that bicarbonate excretion is increased, but this effect is generally small compared with the effect on chloride excretion and does not appreciably alter the pH of the urine. They may also reduce the glomerular filtration rate.

Thiazide diuretics reduce circulating fluid volume that reduces the preload on the heart. Cardiac output is therefore reduced, as is blood pressure. When thiazides are given long-term, homeostatic mechanisms come into play (vasodilatation and therefore reduced peripheral vascular resistance) that return cardiac output to normal levels. Thiazide diuretics also have some direct vasodilatory properties and enhance the effects of other antihypertensive drugs.

For thiazide diuretics to act they must be delivered in the urine to their site of action on the tubular epithelium. Most thiazide diuretics are ineffective in patients with renal impairment who have a creatinine clearance of less than 30 ml/min since not enough of the drug is delivered to its site of action.

Thiazide diuretics have been extensively tested in large clinical trials and have shown clear reductions in incidence of stroke (by about 40%). In the early trials, the reduction in coronary heart disease was disappointing but this may have been due to the large doses that were formerly used causing adverse metabolic effects. More recent trials that have used lower doses have produced much larger reductions in coronary heart disease, especially in the elderly.

There is little to choose between the various thiazide diuretics available (see Table 7.1).

Pharmacokinetics[1]

Thiazide and related diuretics vary considerably in their pharmacokinetics. Most are highly bound to either plasma proteins or red blood cells or both. Some (bendroflumethiazide (bendrofluazide), indapamide) undergo fairly extensive metabolism and others are excreted largely unchanged (chlortalidone, hydrochlorothiazide; see Table 7.1).

Dosage

See Table 7.1.

Thiazide diuretics are usually given in the morning so that sleep is not interrupted by diuresis. Diuresis is initiated in about 1–2 h

Table 7.1 Thiazide and related diuretics

Thiazide diuretic	Half-life (h)	Duration of effect (h)	Daily dose	Tablet strength (mg)	Comments	Proprietary name(s) (UK)	Manufacturer(s) (UK)
Bendroflumethiazide (bendrofluazide)	3–4	12–18	2.5 mg	2.5 and 5		Aprinox, Berkozide, Neo-Bendromax, Neo-NaClex	APS, Ashbourne, Berk, Cox, Goldshield, Hillcross, Norton, Sovereign
Chlortalidone	40–60	48–72	25 mg, increased to 50 µg if necessary	50		Hygroton	Alliance
Cyclopenthiazide		12	Initially 250 mg increased to 500 µg if necessary	500 µg		Navidrex	Alliance
Hydrochlorothiazide	5–15	6–12	25 mg, increased to 50 mg if necessary	25 and 50	In some patients (especially the elderly) an initial dose of 12.5 mg may be sufficient	HydroSaluric	MSD

Table 7.1 Contd.

Thiazide diuretic	Half-life (h)	Duration of effect (h)	Daily dose	Tablet strength (mg)	Comments	Proprietary name(s) (UK)	Manufacturer(s) (UK)
Indapamide	14		2.5 mg	2.5	Modified-release preparation available (different dose)	Natramid, Natrilix, Nindaxa 2.5, Opumide	APS, Ashbourne, Cox, Hillcross, Norton, Opus, Servier, Sterwin, Trinity
Metolazone	4–5 (in plasma) 8–10 (in whole blood)	12–24	5 mg initially; maintenance 5 mg on alternate days	5	In some countries a preparation with enhanced bioavailability is available that is used in a lower dose	Metenix 5	Borg
Polythiazide	26	24–48	Usually 1–4 mg	1	0.5 mg may be adequate in some patients	Nephril	Pfizer
Xipamide	5–8	12	20 mg	20		Diurexan	ASTA Medica

following the oral administration of most thiazides and most have a duration of action of about 12–24 h.

The dosage of thiazide diuretics should be adjusted to the minimum effective dose, especially in the elderly, and in recent years there has been a definite trend towards lower doses.[2] They tend to produce a maximal response on blood pressure at relatively low doses and further increases in dose simply increase side-effects with little further effect on blood pressure. The maximum therapeutic effect may not be evident for several weeks.

Adverse effects[3]

Thiazide diuretics may cause a number of metabolic disturbances, especially at high doses, and their use can result in electrolyte imbalances.[4] These adverse effects cause thiazides to be contraindicated in certain diseases or conditions (see Adverse Effects Focus, below).

ADVERSE EFFECTS FOCUS

Contraindications for thiazide therapy

- Addison's disease
- Severe renal impairment/anuria (thiazides are not effective in patients with a creatinine clearance of <30 ml/min) – may be used with caution in less severe renal impairment but there is the risk of further reduction in renal function
- Severe hepatic impairment – encephalopathy may be precipitated
- Pre-existing hypercalcaemia
- Symptomatic hyperuricaemia (history of gout or uric acid calculi)

Effects on electrolytes

Due to their effects on electrolyte absorption in the distal tubule, administration of thiazide diuretics may be associated with various electrolyte imbalances, including hypochloraemic alkalosis, hyponatraemia and hypokalaemia. They should therefore be used with caution in patients with existing fluid and electrolyte disturbances or who are at risk from changes in fluid and electrolyte balance, such as the elderly. The dose should be carefully adjusted according to renal function and clinical response in the elderly. Thiazides should be used with caution in patients with impaired hepatic function or progressive liver disease, since minor alterations of fluid and electrolyte balance may precipitate hepatic coma. All patients should be carefully observed for signs of fluid and electrolyte imbalance (see Adverse Effects Focus, below).

ADVERSE EFFECTS FOCUS

Patients at risk of electrolyte imbalance (regular monitoring of serum and urine electrolyte concentrations is recommended)

- Excessive vomiting
- During parenteral fluid therapy
- Elderly
- Ascites due to liver cirrhosis
- Oedema due to nephrotic syndrome
- Digitalised patients

Hypokalaemia

Thiazide diuretics can cause hypokalaemia. Hypokalaemia intensifies the effect of digitalis on cardiac muscle and can cause adverse drug effects in patients taking other drugs that prolong the QT interval on the electrocardiogram (ECG; see p. 66). A major concern has been that thiazide-induced hypokalaemia might predispose to cardiac arrhythmias and sudden cardiac death. However, studies looking at the possible association have produced conflicting results. Patients with cirrhosis of the liver are particularly at risk from hypokalaemia. If hypokalaemia is accompanied by clinical signs, the thiazide must be discontinued.

Potassium stores may be maintained either by concurrent use of a potassium-sparing diuretic such as amiloride or triamterene (see Chapter 13) or, less commonly, by administration of potassium supplements. Foods with a high potassium content such as milk, bananas and raisins may help maintain potassium levels, as may moderate sodium restriction. However, routine potassium supplementation or conservation is not necessary[5] unless the serum potassium concentration falls below 3.0 mmol/l. It is more likely to be needed in those particularly at risk from the cardiac effects of hypokalaemia, such as those taking digitalis or with severe liver disease.[6] The risk of hypokalaemia is greatest at high doses, in the elderly, in patients with other chronic debilitating illness and when patients take other drugs which promote potassium loss (see p. 66).

Hyponatraemia

Diuretic therapy is a common cause of hyponatraemia. It may occur particularly in patients with severe heart failure who are very oedematous, especially if they are taking large doses of thiazides in conjunction with restricted salt in the diet. The elderly also appear to be particularly susceptible, possibly because of inappropriate secretion of antidiuretic hormone.[7] It has been suggested that hyponatraemia may be more likely in patients taking a combination of hydrochlorothiazide with a potassium-sparing diuretic.[8,9]

Hypercalcaemia

The urinary excretion of calcium is reduced by thiazides and can sometimes result in mild hypercalcaemia; thiazide diuretics should not be given to patients with pre-existing hypercalcaemia. Hypertension is a complication of primary hyperparathyroidism and thiazide diuretics have often been withheld in these patients for fear of exacerbating hypercalcaemia. However, studies have not confirmed that this is a problem and thiazide diuretics are not contraindicated in such patients. They should however be stopped before parathyroid function is tested.

Hypomagnesaemia

Hypomagnesaemia has occurred; as with hypokalaemia (above), it has been implicated as a risk factor for cardiac arrhythmias.

Signs of electrolyte imbalance

Warning signs of electrolyte imbalance include dry mouth, thirst, weakness, lethargy, drowsiness, restlessness, confusion, tachycardia, muscle pain and cramps, seizures, oliguria, hypotension and gastrointestinal disturbances such as nausea and vomiting. All patients should be carefully observed for signs of fluid and electrolyte imbalance. Certain situations need closer monitoring (see Adverse Effects Focus, p. 63).

Effects on carbohydrates and lipids

Thiazide diuretics can increase serum low-density lipoprotein (LDL)-cholesterol, very-low-density lipoprotein (VLDL)-cholesterol and triglyceride levels and there is concern that these adverse lipid changes may offset the beneficial effects of lowering the blood pressure. It appears that these changes to lipids may not persist long-term[10] and it has been argued that changes are likely to be slight with the low doses now used for treating hypertension. However, the concerns remain in some quarters.

Thiazide diuretics can provoke hyperglycaemia and glycosuria in diabetic and other susceptible patients and, rarely, have precipitated frank diabetes. However, again, this appears to be a dose-related effect and is much less likely with the low doses now used. If thiazide diuretics are used in patients taking antidiabetics, blood glucose concentrations should be monitored, since requirements may change (see p. 66).

To summarise, although thiazide diuretics should probably be avoided as first-line drugs in patients with diabetes and those with hyperlipidaemia, there should be no anxiety about adding them in where necessary.

Hyperuricaemia

Thiazide diuretics may cause hyperuricaemia and precipitate attacks of gout in some patients even at low doses.

Other side-effects

Thiazide diuretics can cause various gastrointestinal effects such as anorexia, gastric irritation, nausea, vomiting, constipation and diarrhoea. Other side-effects include headache, dizziness, photosensitivity reactions, postural hypotension, paraesthesia and yellow vision. Impotence may occasionally be a problem.

Hypersensitivity reactions, including skin rashes, fever, pulmonary oedema and pneumonitis, have occurred. Cholestatic jaundice, pancreatitis and blood dyscrasias, including thrombocytopenia and, more rarely, granulocytopenia, leukopenia and aplastic and haemolytic anaemia have been reported.

Intestinal ulceration has occurred following the administration of tablets containing thiazides with an enteric-coated core of potassium chloride. Thiazide diuretics may exacerbate or activate systemic lupus erythematosus in susceptible patients.

Drug interactions[11]

The antihypertensive effect of thiazides and related diuretics is enhanced by concomitant administration with other drugs that have a secondary hypotensive effect and antagonised by administration with other drugs that have a hypertensive effect (see Chapter 16).

Many of the interactions of thiazide diuretics are due to their effects on fluid and electrolyte balance.

Hypokalaemia-induced interactions

Diuretic-induced hypokalaemia may enhance the toxicity of digitalis glycosides and administration of glycosides may have to be temporarily suspended. Hypokalaemia may also increase the risk of cardiac arrhythmias with drugs that prolong the QT interval on ECG; such drugs include astemizole, halofantrine, pimozide, sotalol and terfenadine.

Thiazide-induced hypokalaemia probably also explains the interaction of thiazide diuretics with competitive muscle relaxants, such as tubocurarine; use of the combination may produce enhanced neuromuscular blockade.

Hypokalaemic effect enhanced

A more pronounced potassium-depleting effect may be produced if thiazide diuretics are given concurrently with amphotericin, carbenoxolone, corticosteroids, corticotropin or $beta_2$ agonists such as salbutamol.

Hypotensive effect enhanced

Thiazide diuretics enhance the effect of most other antihypertensives given concomitantly and this is used to beneficial effect in the management of hypertension. However, certain combinations should be introduced cautiously. For example, thiazide diuretics may enhance the first-dose hypotension that occurs with alpha blockers or ACE inhibitors. Thiazide diuretics should be discontinued or the dose significantly reduced 2–3 days before the initiation of treatment with an ACE inhibitor. Postural hypotension associated with diuretic therapy may be enhanced by concomitant ingestion of alcohol, barbiturates or opioids.

Hypotensive effect antagonised

Drugs that cause fluid retention, such as carbenoxolone, corticosteroids or NSAIDs (see Chapter 16) may antagonise the hypotensive effect of thiazide diuretics.

Allopurinol

Concurrent use of a thiazide diuretic and allopurinol has produced increased allopurinol toxicity.

Antibacterials

Severe hyponatraemia has been reported in patients taking trimethoprim with co-amilozide (amiloride and hydrochlorothiazide) and hydrochlorothiazide. Increased tetracycline toxicity has been reported when tetracyclines are given concomitantly with thiazide diuretics.

Anticoagulants

Chlortalidone has been associated with a reduction in the activity of warfarin in healthy subjects. It has been suggested that this might be a consequence of the diuresis concentrating the circulating clotting factors.

Antidiabetics

Thiazide diuretics may alter requirements for hypoglycaemic drugs in diabetic patients.

Antiepileptics

Symptomatic hyponatraemia has been reported with concomitant use of hydrochlorothiazide and carbamazepine.

Bile acid binding resins

Colestyramine and colestipol have been reported to reduce significantly the gastrointestinal absorption of hydrochlorothiazide. Separating administration by as much as 4 hours still reduced absorption.

Calcium salts[12]

Concomitant administration of calcium carbonate in moderately large doses together with a thiazide diuretic has led to the development of the milk-alkali syndrome (characterised by hypercalcaemia, metabolic alkalosis and renal failure). Thiazide diuretics reduce the excretion of calcium and therefore patients taking thiazide diuretics in combination with calcium salts may be at increased risk of developing the milk-alkali syndrome. Hypercalcaemia may also occur in patients taking thiazide diuretics with drugs that increase calcium levels, such as vitamin D.

Ciclosporin

Concomitant treatment with ciclosporin and a thiazide diuretic may increase the risk of hyperuricaemia and gout-type complications. Addition of a thiazide in a patient already taking ciclosporin has increased ciclosporin-induced nephrotoxicity.

Dopaminergics

Initiation of treatment with triamterene and hydrochlorothiazide in a patient established on amantadine therapy was associated with development of amantadine toxicity; reduction of tubular secretion of amantadine was considered a possible cause.

Lithium

Thiazide diuretics should not usually be administered concomitantly with lithium since the association may lead to toxic blood concentrations of lithium. If the combination must be used, the dose of lithium should be reduced and lithium concentrations measured frequently until they re-stabilise.[13]

Pressor amines

Thiazide diuretics have been reported to diminish the response to pressor amines, such as noradrenaline (norepinephrine), but the clinical significance of this effect is uncertain.

Preparations

See Table 7.1.

References

1. Welling P G. Pharmacokinetics of the thiazide diuretics. *Biopharm Drug Dispos* 1986; 7: 501–535.
2. Ramsay L E. Thiazide diuretics in hypertension. *Clin Exp Hypertens* 1999; 21: 805–814.
3. Greenberg A. Diuretic complications. *Am J Med Sci* 2000; 319: 10–24.
4. Ramsay L E, Yeo W W, Jackson P R. Metabolic effects of diuretics. *Cardiology* 1994; 84 (suppl 2): 48–56.
5. Anonymous. Routine use of potassium-sparing diuretics. *Drug Ther Bull* 1992; 29: 85–87.
6. Anonymous. Potassium-sparing diuretics – when are they really needed? *Drug Ther Bull* 1985; 23: 17–20.
7. Sonnenblick M, Algur N, Rosin A. Thiazide-induced hyponatremia and vasopressin release. *Ann Intern Med* 1989; 110: 751.
8. Roberts C J C, Channer K S, Bungay D. Hyponatraemia induced by a combination of hydrochlorothiazide and triamterene. *BMJ* 1984; 288: 1962.
9. Millson D, Borland C, Murphy P, Davison W. Hyponatraemia and Moduretic (amiloride plus hydrochlorothiazide). *BMJ* 1984; 289: 1308–1309.
10. Grimm R H, Flack J M, Grandits G A. Long-term effects on plasma lipids of diet and drugs used to treat hypertension. *JAMA* 1996; 275: 1549–1556.
11. Stockley I H. *Drug Interactions*, 5th edn. London: Pharmaceutical Press, 1999.
12. Gora M L, Seth S K, Bay W H, Visconti J A. Milk-alkali syndrome associated with use of chlorothiazide and calcium carbonate. *Clin Pharm* 1989; 8: 227–229.
13. Beeley L. Drug interactions with lithium. *Prescribers' J* 1986; 26: 160–163.

8

Beta blockers

Indications

Beta blockers are first-choice agents in hypertension. They are particularly recommended for those patients who have suffered a myocardial infarction. They tend to be less effective in black patients.

Beta blockers may be used in combination with other antihypertensives. Combination with a thiazide is common.

Mechanism of action

Beta blockers (also known as beta-adrenoceptor blocking drugs or antagonists) were introduced in 1965, originally for the management of angina. Beta blockers block the action of noradrenaline (norepinephrine) at beta-adrenoceptors and their major effect is to slow the heart rate and reduce the force of contraction. It is not completely understood how they act in hypertension: possible mechanisms include reduced cardiac output, altered baroreceptor reflex sensitivity, blockade of peripheral adrenoceptors, reduced plasma renin secretion or a central effect.[1] Stimulation of vasodilator prostaglandins and increase in atrial natriuretic factor have also been proposed.

Many beta blockers are available (see Figure 8.1 and Table 8.1) and in general they are all equally effective in reducing blood pressure, although individual beta blockers differ according to their pharmacological properties (see below) and these differences may affect choice in treating individual patients.

The main method for characterising beta blockers is according to their affinity for the two subtypes of beta-adrenergic receptor, $beta_1$ and $beta_2$. $Beta_1$ receptors are found mainly in the heart and blockade of these receptors reduces heart rate, myocardial contractility and the rate of conduction of impulses through the conducting system. Blockade of $beta_1$ receptors also produces suppression of adrenergic-induced renin release and lipolysis. $Beta_2$ receptors are found in non-cardiac tissue, including bronchial tissue and peripheral blood vessels.

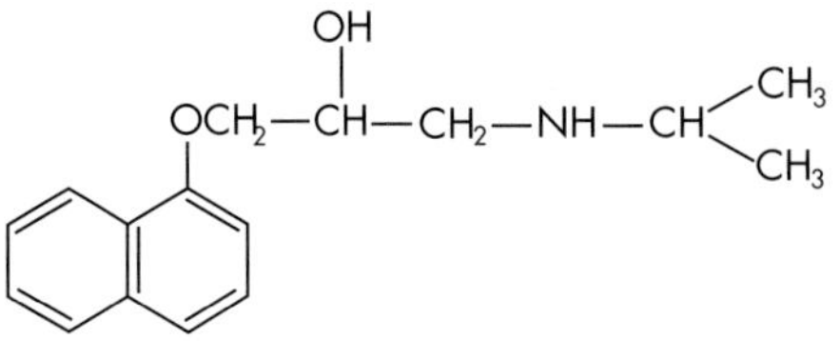

Propranolol – non-selective

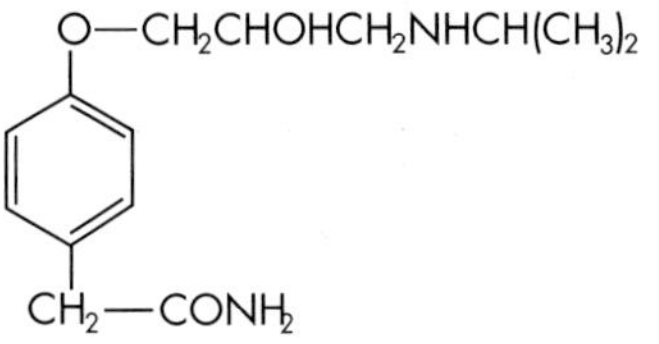

Atenolol – cardioselective

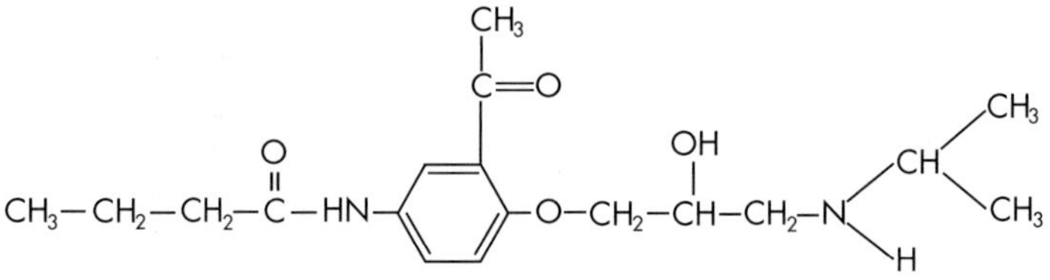

Acebutolol – intrinsic sympathomimetic activity

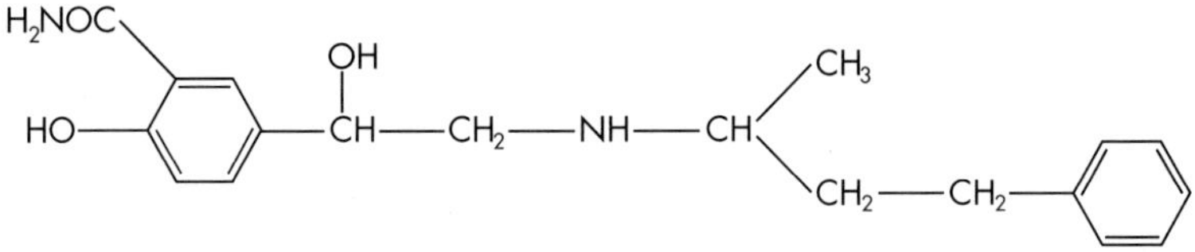

Labetalol – alpha blocking activity

Figure 8.1 Beta blockers.

Blockade of these receptors produces increased bronchial resistance and inhibition of catecholamine-induced glucose metabolism. $Beta_2$ receptors may also have a role in the regulation of heart rate. It is now recognised that in some organs, including the heart, both receptor sub-types are present.

Table 8.1 Beta blockers

Beta blocker	Cardio-selectivity	Lipid solubility	ISA	Half-life (h)	Elimination	Daily dose	Tablet strength (mg)	Comments	Proprietary name(s) (UK)	Manufacturer(s) (UK)
Acebutolol	Yes	Low to moderate	Moderate	3–4 (acebutolol), 8–13 (diacetolol, active metabolite)	Extensively metabolised (active metabolite); excreted in urine and bile	400 mg initially increased after 2 weeks if necessary to 800 mg (in two divided doses)	100, 200 and 400	Acebutolol and active metabolite both removed by dialysis. Half-lives increased in the elderly and in renal impairment	Sectral	Akita
Atenolol	Yes	Low	Absent/low	6–7	Little/no metabolism; excreted in urine	50 mg	25, 50 and 100	Reduced doses may be needed in renal impairment	Antipressan, Atenix, Tenormin	Antigen, APS, Ashbourne, AstraZeneca, Berk, Cox, CP, Hillcross, Norton, Sterwin, Tillomed
Betaxolol hydrochloride	Yes	High	Absent/low	16–20	Metabolised: excreted in urine	20 mg increased to 40 mg if necessary	20	10 mg in elderly. Reduce dose in severe renal impairment	Kerlone	Sanofi-Synthelabo
Bisoprolol fumarate	Yes	Moderate	Absent/low	10–12	About 50% metabolised; excreted in urine	10 mg daily; max. 20 mg	5 and 10	5 mg may be adequate in some patients	Emcor, Monocor	Lederle, Merck
Carvedilol	No	High	Absent/low	6–10	Extensively metabolised; excreted mainly in bile	12.5 mg initially, increased after 2 days to 25 mg; may be increased at intervals of at least 2 weeks to max. 50 mg (in single or divided doses)	3.125, 6.25, 12.5 and 25	Initial dose of 12.5 mg daily may be adequate in elderly. Also has vasodilating activity attributed to alpha$_1$ blocking action. Not recommended in hepatic dysfunction	Eucardic	Roche

continued overleaf

Table 8.1 Contd.

Beta blocker	Cardio-selectivity	Lipid solubility	ISA	Half-life (h)	Elimination	Daily dose	Tablet strength (mg)	Comments	Proprietary name(s) (UK)	Manufacturer(s) (UK)
Celiprolol hydrochloride	Yes	Low	Moderate	5–6	Minimal metabolism; excreted in urine and bile	200 mg increased to 400 mg if necessary	200 and 400	Give in the morning. Has direct vasodilator activity. Reduced doses may be needed in renal impairment	Celectol	Generics, Norton, Pantheon
Labetalol hydrochloride	No	Low	Absent/low	8	Metabolised; excreted in urine, some in bile	200 mg initially (elderly 100 mg), increased at intervals of 14 days to usual dose of 400 mg; max. 2.4 g	50, 100, 200 and 400	Give with food. Daily dose given in two divided doses (3–4 divided doses if more than 800 mg daily). Severe hepatocellular damage has been reported with short- and long-term use. Also possesses alpha$_1$ blocking activity, therefore postural hypotension may occur at start of treatment or with high doses	Trandate	Cox, Hillcross, Medeva, Norton
Metoprolol tartrate	Yes	Moderate	Absent/low	3–4 (fast hydroxylators); 7 (poor hydroxylators)	Extensively metabolised (rate determined by genetic polymorphism); excreted in urine	100 mg initially; maintenance 100–200 mg (in 1–2 divided doses)	50 and 100	Modified-release preparations also available. Reduce dose in hepatic impairment	Betaloc, Lopresor, Mepranix	APS, Ashbourne, AstraZeneca, Cox, Hillcross, Norton, Novartis

Table 8.1 Contd.

Beta blocker	Cardio-selectivity	Lipid solubility	ISA	Half-life (h)	Elimination	Daily dose	Tablet strength (mg)	Comments	Proprietary name(s) (UK)	Manufacturer(s) (UK)
Nadolol	No	Low	Absent/low	12–24	Not metabolised; excreted in urine	80 mg increased at weekly intervals if necessary to max. 240 mg	40 and 80	Dialysable. Reduced doses may be needed in renal impairment	Corgard	Sanofi-Synthelabo
Nebivolol	Yes		Absent/low			5 mg (2.5 mg initially in elderly)	5	Has vasodilating activity	Nebilet	Menarini
Oxprenolol hydrochloride	No	Moderate	Moderate	1–2	Metabolised; excreted in urine	80–160 mg (in 2–3 divided doses); max. 320 mg	20, 40, 80 and 160	Modified-release preparations also available	Trasicor	Hillcross, Norton, Novartis
Pindolol	No	Moderate	High	3–4	Partially metabolised; excreted in urine	10–15 mg initially (as single dose or 2–3 divided doses) increased if necessary at weekly intervals; usual maintenance 15–30 mg; max. 45 mg	5 and 15	Half-life prolonged in elderly, or in renal, or hepatic impairment	Visken	Novartis
Propranolol hydrochloride	No	High	Absent/low	3–6	Extensively metabolised; excreted in urine	160 mg initially (in two divided doses) increased at weekly intervals as required; maintenance 160–320 mg	10, 40, 80 and 160	Not dialysed. Modified-release preparations also available	Angilol, Inderal, Propanix	Ashbourne, AstraZeneca, Cox, DDSA, Hillcross
Timolol maleate	No	Low to moderate	Absent/low	4	Extensively metabolised; excreted in urine	10 mg initially (as single dose or two divided doses) increased if necessary to max. 60 mg	10	Daily doses over 20 mg should be given as divided doses. Reduced doses may be needed in renal or hepatic impairment	Betim	Leo

ISA = Intrinsic sympathomimetic activity.

Beta blockers that act principally on beta$_1$ receptors (such as atenolol and metoprolol) are known as cardioselective agents. They have less action on beta$_2$ receptors in the bronchi and peripheral vessels compared with non-selective agents, such as oxprenolol and propranolol, and therefore beta$_2$ receptor-mediated side-effects (such as bronchospasm and effects on carbohydrate and lipid metabolism, see Adverse effects, p. 78) are reduced. It is important to note that these beta$_2$ receptor effects are not abolished completely. Their selectivity is only relative and, as doses are increased, activity at beta$_2$ receptors becomes clinically important.

Beta blockers may also be characterised by the presence of intrinsic sympathomimetic activity, blockade of alpha-adrenergic receptors, and membrane-stabilising activity (see Table 8.1).

Beta blockers with intrinsic sympathomimetic activity (also known as partial agonist activity), for example, acebutolol, celiprolol, oxprenolol and pindolol, stimulate beta receptors when background sympathetic nervous activity is low and block them when activity is high. This activity produces less resting bradycardia and possibly fewer problems with cold extremities than other beta blockers. However, in practice, they are little used in the treatment of hypertension.

Beta blockers that also block alpha-adrenergic receptors (carvedilol and labetalol) produce a reduction in peripheral vascular resistance in addition to their effect of slowing the heart rate. However, such agents have the disadvantage of possessing the side-effects of both classes of drug. In addition to its beta$_1$-blocking activities, carvedilol also has antioxidant effects, which give it theoretical advantages in reducing endothelial damage and lowering levels of highly atherogenic oxidised low-density lipoprotein (LDL)-cholesterol.

At high blood concentrations, propranolol and some other beta blockers also possess a membrane-stabilising effect. This effect may not be evident at therapeutic doses but may be important in overdose.

Other beta blockers, such as celiprolol, also have vasodilator properties that may be due to various mechanisms, including alpha$_1$ blockade, beta$_2$ stimulation and direct vasodilator activity.

Contraindications

Due to some of the side-effects of beta blockers, beta blockers are contraindicated in the presence of certain conditions (see Adverse Effects Focus, p. 77). Special caution is required if beta blockers are used in patients with diabetes (see p. 79). Beta blockers may mask symptoms of hyperthyroidism such as tachycardia. Caution is needed in patients with

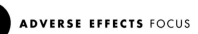

ADVERSE EFFECTS FOCUS

Contraindications for beta blocker therapy
• Metabolic acidosis • Second- and third-degree heart block • Uncontrolled heart failure • Bronchospasm/asthma/history of obstructive airways disease (see p. 78) • Severe peripheral vascular disease • Prinzmetal's angina (may increase the number and duration of attacks – a cardioselective beta blocker may be considered but extreme caution is necessary) • Bradycardia (less than 45–50 beats/min – but see p. 78) • Cardiogenic shock

a history of anaphylaxis to an antigen since these patients may be more reactive to repeated challenge with the antigen while taking beta blockers. Also beta blockers may reduce responsiveness to adrenaline (epinephrine) used to treat the anaphylactic reactions (see p. 83).

Beta blockers should not be given to patients with phaeochromocytoma without concomitant alpha-adrenoceptor blocking therapy.

Pharmacokinetics[2,3]

Beta blockers differ widely in their pharmacokinetic properties. Differences in lipid solubility are largely responsible for these variations (see Table 8.1). Generally, those with low lipid solubility (e.g. atenolol, celiprolol, nadolol) tend to be less readily absorbed from the gastrointestinal tract and less extensively metabolised, to have low plasma-protein binding and relatively long plasma half-lives, and to cross the blood–brain barrier less readily than beta blockers with high lipid solubility (e.g. betaxolol, carvedilol, propranolol). The low-lipid-solubility beta blockers are mostly excreted unchanged in the urine, whereas the beta blockers with high lipid solubility are extensively metabolised. These differences need to be borne in mind when choosing a beta blocker for a particular patient and influence whether dose reductions are needed in renal or hepatic impairment (see Table 8.1). There is no clear correlation between plasma concentrations of beta blockers and therapeutic activity, especially when the beta blocker undergoes metabolism to active metabolites (such as acebutolol).

Dosage

See Table 8.1.

Adverse effects[4]

Most of the side-effects of beta blockers are predictable from their mode of action. The most frequent and serious adverse effects of beta blockers are related to their beta-adrenergic blocking activity. The most important side-effects in clinical usage are impaired effort tolerance (most commonly with non-selective beta blockers), cold peripheries and bronchoconstriction.

Cardiovascular effects

Cardiovascular effects include bradycardia and hypotension; heart failure or heart block may be precipitated in patients with underlying cardiac disorders. Sinus bradycardia is common in patients taking beta blockers since heart rate is reduced as a result of the pharmacological action of the drug. It is not in itself a reason to stop the beta blocker. However, rarely, patients develop symptoms and the dose of beta blocker should be reduced in these patients. It should be stopped completely if the heart rate falls below 40 beats/min. Abrupt withdrawal of beta blockers may exacerbate angina and can cause angina, myocardial infarction, ventricular arrhythmias and sudden death. Withdrawal of beta blockers therefore needs to be gradual (over 1–2 weeks in patients who have been on long-term beta blocker therapy), especially in patients with ischaemic heart disease. Reduced peripheral circulation can produce coldness of the extremities and may exacerbate peripheral vascular disease such as Raynaud's syndrome. Nevertheless, they are reasonably tolerated in those with lesser degrees of peripheral vascular disease.[5]

Bronchospasm

Beta blockers can precipitate bronchospasm in susceptible patients due to blockade of beta$_2$ receptors in bronchial smooth muscle. Beta$_1$-selective beta blockers or those that possess intrinsic sympathomimetic activity at beta$_2$ receptors may be less likely to induce bronchospasm, although all beta blockers are contraindicated in patients with bronchospasm, asthma or a history of obstructive airways disease. When there is no alternative to beta blocker treatment in such patients some authorities consider that a cardioselective beta blocker might be used with extreme caution. If bronchospasm occurs it can usually be reversed by giving a beta$_2$ agonist such as salbutamol. Large doses may be required to overcome the beta blockade and it may be necessary to use both the inhalational and intravenous routes. Intravenous aminophylline and nebulised ipratropium may also be considered. Severe cases may require oxygen and artificial ventilation.

Effects on carbohydrate and lipid metabolism

The adrenergic system is involved in the control of carbohydrate and lipid metabolism. Both hypoglycaemia and hyperglycaemia have been reported with the use of beta blockers. In patients with type 1 diabetes mellitus, beta blockade (mediated via beta$_2$ receptors) may mask the adrenaline (epinephrine)-mediated symptoms of hypoglycaemia such as tachycardia and tremor. Beta blockade may also delay recovery from hypoglycaemia in glucose-treated patients. Because of these effects the use of beta blockers in patients who suffer frequent episodes of hypo-glycaemia is best avoided. However, these effects should not prevent their use in patients whose diabetes is well controlled.[6] A beta$_1$-selective (cardioselective) beta blocker, possibly with little or no lipophilicity,[7] such as atenolol, may be preferable for such patients. Regular monitor-ing is required when treatment with the beta blocker is started or when dose adjustments are made. The dose of the antidiabetic should be adjusted as necessary during this period. It is important to ensure that the patient is aware that some of the early warning signs of hypo-glycaemia may not occur.

Effects of beta blockade on lipid metabolism include raised plasma concentrations of very-low-density lipoprotein and triglyceride and reduced plasma concentrations of high-density lipoprotein. These effects have obviously caused much concern as they would be contributing to a patient's level of cardiovascular risk and thus possibly negating the beneficial effects of beta blockers on blood pressure. Beta$_1$-selective (car-dioselective) beta blockers may have less pronounced effects on lipids, as may beta blockers that also possess intrinsic sympathomimetic activity[8] or that also block alpha-adrenergic receptors.

Other side-effects

Other side-effects include central nervous system effects of depression, dizziness, hallucinations, confusion and sleep disturbances, including nightmares. Beta blockers which are lipid-soluble are more likely to enter the brain and would be expected to be associated with a higher incidence of central nervous system adverse effects, although this is not proven.

Fatigue is a common side-effect experienced with beta blockers. Paraesthesia, peripheral neuropathy and myopathies, including muscle cramps, have been reported. Rarely, a myasthenia gravis-like syndrome or exacerbation of myasthenia gravis has been reported. Decreased tear production, blurred vision and soreness are among ocular symptoms which have been reported and can be especially troublesome in wearers of contact lenses, particularly soft lenses. Adverse gastrointestinal effects include nausea and vomiting, diarrhoea, constipation and abdominal cramping.

Skin rash, pruritus and reversible alopecia have occurred with use of beta blockers. Psoriasis may be aggravated.

Other side-effects include a lupus-like syndrome, male impotence, sclerosing peritonitis, retroperitoneal fibrosis, pneumonitis, pulmonary fibrosis, and pleurisy and various haematological reactions.

Drug interactions[9]

Many of the interactions of beta blockers can be predicted on the basis of their effects at beta$_1$ and beta$_2$ receptors.[10,11] Thus, interactions may occur with drugs that interfere with a beta blocker's antihypertensive effect, cardiodepressant effect, effect on carbohydrate metabolism, or effect on bronchial beta$_2$ receptors (see below). The characteristics of the individual beta blocker must therefore be borne in mind when considering likely interactions. See Chapter 16 for possible interactions that may occur with other drugs that have secondary hypotensive or hypertensive effects, including non-steroidal anti-inflammatory drugs (NSAIDs).

Pharmacokinetic interactions may occur with many drugs that alter absorption of beta blockers. For example, aluminium salts and bile acid binding resins, such as cholestyramine, reduce absorption. Pharmacokinetic interactions may also occur with drugs that alter metabolism of beta blockers, such as stimulators of liver enzymes (e.g. phenobarbital and rifampicin) and inhibitors of liver enzymes (e.g. cimetidine and erythromycin). While these interactions may alter the plasma concentration of the beta blocker, they are not usually clinically significant since there is no association between plasma concentrations and therapeutic effect or toxicity and there are wide interindividual differences in steady-state plasma concentrations of beta blockers.

Anaesthetics

Special care is needed in patients on beta blockers who undergo surgery and awareness by the anaesthetist that beta blockers are being taken is of the greatest importance. Beta blockers attenuate the reflex tachycardia that occurs with anaesthetics and increase the risk of hypotension and some have suggested that beta blockers should be withdrawn before anaesthesia. However, this makes the blood pressure unstable and difficult to control during anaesthesia and some anaesthetists prefer the patient to continue taking the beta blocker. In these cases and in emergency surgery the effects of beta blockers may be reversed by an agent such as atropine that counters the increase in vagal tone. Such patients may still be subject to severe protracted hypotension. Anaesthetics that cause myocardial depression, such as ether, cyclopropane and trichloroethylene, should preferably be avoided in patients on beta blockers.

For a warning about use of local anaesthetics, see p. 83.

Antiarrhythmics

Use of beta blockers concomitantly with antiarrhythmic drugs and other drugs that also affect cardiac conduction can precipitate bradycardia and heart block.

Antidepressants

Bradycardia and heart block, occurring shortly after the introduction of treatment with fluoxetine, have been reported in patients receiving metoprolol and propranolol. Impaired conduction through the atrioventricular node and inhibition by fluoxetine of the oxidative metabolism of beta blockers are possible mechanisms. Tricylic antidepressants also have a hypotensive effect and this may potentiate the antihypertensive effect of beta blockers.

Antidiabetics

In diabetic patients beta blockers can modify the response to insulin and oral hypoglycaemics through their effects on pancreatic $beta_2$ receptors (see p. 79).

Antihypertensives

Concurrent use of beta blockers with other antihypertensive drugs produces an enhanced antihypertensive effect that is usually beneficial. However, some combinations should be avoided (see Calcium-channel blockers, below). Beta blockers can potentiate the severe postural hypotension that may follow the initial dose of prazosin. Beta blockers may exacerbate rebound hypertension following withdrawal of clonidine treatment; clonidine should not be withdrawn until several days after the withdrawal of the beta blocker.

Antimalarials

Some antimalarials can cause cardiac conduction defects. Such antimalarials include halofantrine, mefloquine and quinine. Cardiopulmonary arrest has occurred after a single dose of mefloquine in a patient taking propranolol.

Calcium-channel blockers

Hypotension, bradycardia, conduction defects and cardiac failure have occurred when calcium-channel blockers and beta blockers have been used concurrently.[12]

The combination of a beta blocker with verapamil (the most cardiodepressant of the calcium-channel blockers) should be particularly avoided. Use of diltiazem, which is less cardiodepressant, with a beta blocker should also be avoided, although some consider they may be used together with caution. Although beta blockers are reportedly safe in combination with the dihydropyridine calcium-channel blockers such as nifedipine, heart failure and severe hypotension have been reported; if the combination is used the blood pressure should be monitored closely, especially during the initial stages of therapy with the combination.

Digoxin

Beta blockers may potentiate bradycardia due to digoxin.

Ergot derivatives

There is an increased risk of peripheral vasoconstriction during concomitant administration of ergotamine and beta blockers. Enhancement of the cardiac-depressant action of propranolol has been reported with concurrent nicergoline use.

Lidocaine (lignocaine)

Administration of propranolol during lidocaine (lignocaine) infusion may increase plasma lidocaine concentration by about 30% and the combination should be avoided. When lidocaine is being used as a local anaesthetic, preparations that include an added vasoconstrictor, such as adrenaline (epinephrine), should be avoided (see below, under Sympathomimetics).

Parasympathomimetics

Bradycardia and hypotension have occurred following the administration of neostigmine or physostigmine to patients receiving beta blockers. Since beta blockers have the potential to aggravate symptoms of myasthenia gravis, they may reduce the effectiveness of treatment with parasympathomimetics.

Sympathomimetics

The effects of sympathomimetics are impaired by blockade of peripheral beta receptors and patients on beta blockers, especially non-selective beta blockers, who are given adrenaline, can develop elevated blood pressure. The bronchodilator effects of adrenaline are also inhibited. Patients on long-term treatment with beta blockers may find that their response to adrenaline given for anaphylaxis is reduced.

Thyroid drugs

Reduced plasma propranolol concentrations have been found in hypothyroid patients receiving long-term treatment with propranolol when treatment with levothyroxine (thyroxine) is started. Propranolol can itself reduce the activity of levothyroxine by inhibiting the deiodination of levothyroxine to tri-iodothyronine, resulting in decreased concentrations of tri-iodothyronine with a concomitant rise in the concentration of inactive reverse tri-iodothyronine.

Preparations

See Table 8.1.

References

1. Hampton J R. Choosing the right β-blocker. *Drugs* 1994; 48: 549–568.
2. Kendall M J. Clinical relevance of pharmacokinetic differences between beta blockers. *Am J Cardiol* 1997; 80: 15J–19J.
3. Borchard U. Pharmacokinetics of beta-adrenoceptor blocking agents: clinical significance of hepatic and/or renal clearance. *Clin Physiol Biochem* 1990; 8 (suppl 2): 28–34.
4. Lewis R V, Lofthouse C. Adverse reactions with beta-adrenoceptor blocking drugs: an update. *Drug Safety* 1993; 9: 272–279.
5. Heintzen M P, Strauer B E. Peripheral vascular effects of beta-blockers. *Eur Heart J* 1994; 15 (suppl C): 2–7.
6. Majumdar S R. Beta-blockers for the treatment of hypertension in patients with diabetes: exploring the contraindication myth. *Cardiovasc Drugs Ther* 1999; 13: 435–439.
7. O'Byrne S, Feely J. Effects of drugs on glucose tolerance in non-insulin-dependent diabetics (part 1). *Drugs* 1990; 40: 6–18.
8. Krone W, Nägele H. Effects of antihypertensives on plasma lipids and lipoprotein metabolism. *Am Heart J* 1988; 116: 1729–1734.
9. Stockley I H. *Drug Interactions*, 5th edn. London: Pharmaceutical Press, 1999.
10. McDevitt D G. Interactions that matter: 12. β-adrenoceptor antagonists. *Prescribers' J* 1988; 28: 25–30.
11. Blaufarb I, Pfeifer T M, Frishman W H. β-Blockers: drug interactions of clinical significance. *Drug Safety* 1995; 13: 359–370.
12. Lam Y W F, Shepherd A M M. Drug interactions in hypertensive patients: pharmacokinetic, pharmacodynamic and genetic considerations. *Clin Pharmacokinet* 1990; 18: 295–317.

9

ACE inhibitors

Indications

Angiotensin-converting enzyme (ACE) inhibitors are alternative first-line agents that may be considered for hypertension when thiazides and beta blockers are contraindicated or not tolerated. They are particularly indicated in patients who also have diabetes, heart failure, or in patients who have left ventricular dysfunction. ACE inhibitors tend to be less effective antihypertensive agents in blacks and in the elderly, who generally have lower renin levels than the general population.

ACE inhibitors may be used as monotherapy or can be usefully combined with a thiazide or a calcium-channel blocker.

Mechanism of action[1]

ACE inhibitors represent one of the major advances in cardiovascular therapeutics over the past 20 years. They were developed after the elucidation of the importance of the renin–angiotensin–aldosterone system in the pathophysiology of hypertension and were introduced into clinical practice in the 1970s. Captopril was the first ACE inhibitor used.

ACE inhibitors are antihypertensive drugs that act by blocking the renin–angiotensin system. They are slow competitive inhibitors of ACE, a peptidyl carboxypeptidase that is present both as a membrane-bound form in endothelial and other cells and as a soluble form in the blood and numerous body fluids (see Figure 9.1). Evidence suggests that inhibition of tissue ACE rather than circulating ACE is the major factor determining haemodynamic effects. ACE catalyses the conversion of the inactive angiotensin I to the powerful vasoconstrictor and stimulator of aldosterone release, angiotensin II (an octapeptide). Inhibition of ACE thus results in vasodilatation, decreased peripheral vascular resistance and a reduction in the levels of the sodium-retaining hormone aldosterone. Plasma renin activity is increased through loss of feedback inhibition. ACE inhibitors have a minimal effect on heart rate. ACE is identical to bradykininase or kininase II, an enzyme that degrades the

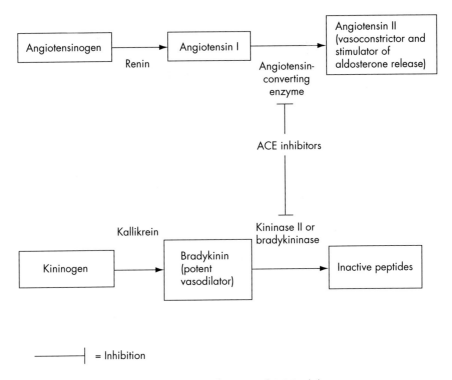

Figure 9.1 Schematic representation of action of ACE inhibitors.

potent vasodilator bradykinin. Inhibition of ACE thus also reduces the degradation of bradykinin and adds to the hypotensive effect of ACE inhibitors, although the increased levels of bradykinin may be responsible for their most troublesome side-effect – cough. ACE inhibitors also produce beneficial effects on renal haemodynamics; they reduce intraglomerular hypertension, resulting in improvements in proteinuric renal disease. ACE inhibitors may affect enzymes involved in the generation of prostaglandins.

ACE inhibitors are usually dipeptide or tripeptide analogues (see Figure 9.2). The active site of ACE has a zinc ion that is important to its catalytic process and ACE inhibitors have generally been designed to bind to this zinc ion. Three chemical groups have been used as zinc ligands: a sulfhydryl group (as in the ACE inhibitor captopril), a carboxyl group (as in enalapril), and a phosphonyl group (as in fosinopril).

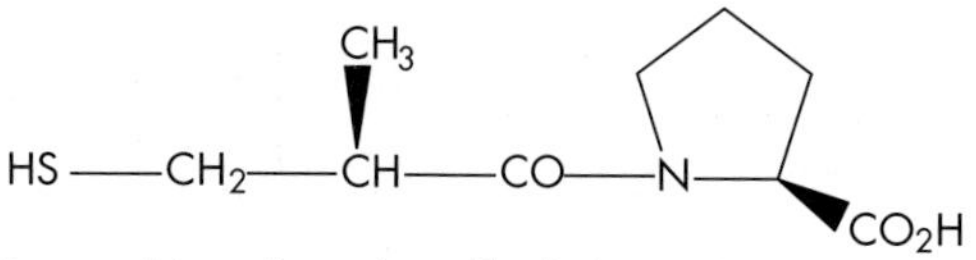

Captopril (zinc ligand – sulfhydryl group)

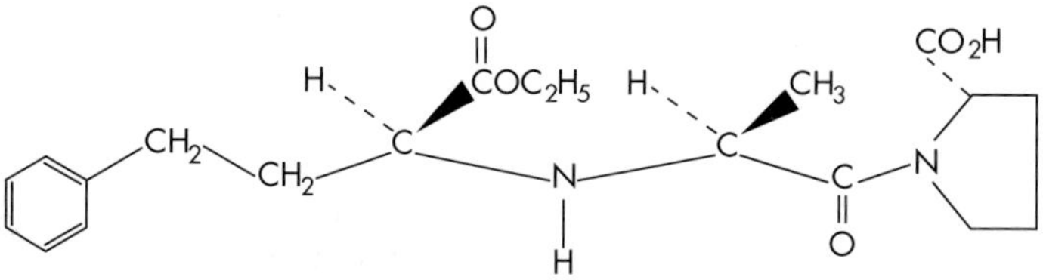

Enalapril (zinc ligand – carboxyl group)

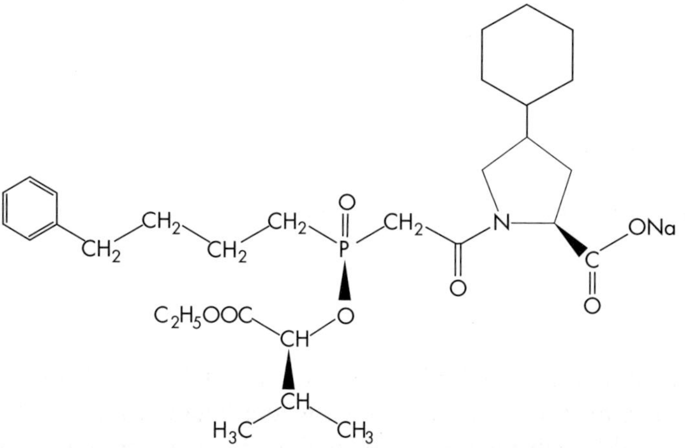

Fosinopril sodium (zinc ligand – phosphonyl group)

Figure 9.2 ACE inhibitors.

Contraindications and precautions

Adverse effects on renal function are a particular concern with ACE inhibitors; see Adverse Effects Focus (p. 88) for the contraindications and cautions to be observed to minimise renal effects. Although some consider renovascular disease to be a contraindication to the use of ACE inhibitors, they may be needed to control blood pressure in some patients. However, they should be used cautiously and in low doses[2] and renal function needs to be monitored with great care.

ADVERSE EFFECTS FOCUS

Precautions to minimise renal adverse effects
• Check renal function in all patients before starting therapy with an ACE inhibitor and monitor regularly during treatment
• Known or suspected renovascular disease – use ACE inhibitors with caution. Renal function must be monitored carefully and reduced doses and/or reduced frequency of doses may be needed
• Severe bilateral renal artery stenosis or severe stenosis of the artery supplying a single functioning kidney: ACE inhibitors are contraindicated or should be used with extreme caution
• Peripheral vascular disease/severe generalised atherosclerosis: ACE inhibitors should be used with caution since such patients could have undiagnosed/clinically silent renovascular disease
• Elderly patients: use ACE inhibitors with caution as these patients are especially at risk of renal side-effects
• Avoid concomitant NSAID use

Hypotension may occur especially at the start of therapy; certain patients are at a particular risk of this adverse effect (see Adverse Effects Focus, p. 89). The first dose of an ACE inhibitor should preferably be given at bedtime to avoid problems with hypotension.

ACE inhibitors should not generally be used in patients with aortic stenosis or outflow tract obstruction as a reduction in blood pressure can aggravate the condition.

ACE inhibitors should be avoided or used with caution in patients with hereditary or idiopathic angioedema or who have had angioedema while taking another ACE inhibitor. Patients with collagen vascular disease and patients who are already taking drugs that cause neutropenia or agranulocytosis (see p. 97) are at increased risk of agranulocytosis or neutropenia if ACE inhibitors are also given, especially if they also have impaired renal function. White cell counts should be monitored both before commencing treatment and regularly thereafter.

ACE inhibitors should not be given to patients on dialysis with high-flux polyacrylonitrile membranes or patients undergoing

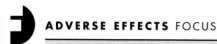

ADVERSE EFFECTS FOCUS

Patients at risk of hypotension

- Those taking concomitant diuretics: discontinue diuretic or significantly reduce the dose for 2–3 days before starting ACE inhibitor
- Dehydrated patients (e.g. following diarrhoea/vomiting)
- Patients with heart failure – if patient is on diuretic, ACE inhibitor must be started under medical supervision for at least 2 h post-dose or until blood pressure has stabilised
- Patients on a low-sodium diet
- Dialysis patients
- Elderly – may be more sensitive to hypotensive effect

low-density lipoprotein apheresis with dextran sulphate as there is an increased risk of anaphylactoid reactions. ACE inhibitors should also be withheld if patients undergo desensitisation with bee or wasp venom as the risk of anaphylactoid reactions is increased.

Pharmacokinetics

Most ACE inhibitors are given by mouth. Food ingestion generally has little effect on absorption. Most ACE inhibitors (captopril and lisinopril are exceptions) are prodrugs and following absorption undergo rapid metabolism by ester hydrolysis (mainly in the liver) to the active diacid form;[3,4] for example, enalapril is converted to enalaprilat. The active drug or active metabolite in most cases is excreted principally in the urine. Some active metabolites, for example fosinoprilat, are also excreted via the biliary tract. ACE inhibitors vary in their binding to plasma proteins. Elimination of the diacid is polyphasic, with a prolonged terminal elimination phase that is considered to represent binding to ACE at a saturable binding site. Since this bound fraction does not contribute to accumulation of drug following multiple doses, an effective half-life for accumulation is usually quoted, as this more accurately predicts the kinetics observed with multiple dosing.

Dosage

See Table 9.1.

Table 9.1 ACE inhibitors

ACE inhibitor	Half-life (h)	Elimination	Prodrug?	Daily dose	Tablet strength (mg)	Comments	Proprietary name(s) (UK)	Manufacturer(s) (UK)
Captopril	2–3	Undergoes some metabolism; excreted in urine (40–50% as unchanged drug)	No	25 mg initially (elderly or with diuretic 12.5 mg); maintenance 50 mg; usual max. 100 mg	12.5, 25 and 50	Removed by dialysis. Daily dose is given in two divided doses	Acepril, Capoten, Ecopace, Hyteneze, Kaplon, Tensopril	Berk, Cox, CP, Galen, Generics, Genus, Goldshield, Hillcross, Lagap, Norton, Opus, Sovereign, Squibb, Sterwin, Tillomed
Cilazapril	9 (cilazaprilat)	Metabolised to cilazaprilat that is excreted unchanged in urine	Yes	1 mg initially (elderly, with a diuretic or in renal impairment 0.5 mg); maintenance 2.5–5 mg; max. 5 mg	0.5, 1, 2.5 and 5	Removed by dialysis	Vascace	Roche

Table 9.1 Contd.

ACE inhibitor	Half-life (h)	Elimination	Prodrug?	Daily dose	Tablet strength (mg)	Comments	Proprietary name(s) (UK)	Manufacturer(s) (UK)
Enalapril maleate	11	Metabolised to enalaprilat that is excreted in urine and faeces	Yes	5 mg initially (elderly, with a diuretic or in renal impairment 2.5 mg); usual maintenance 10–20 mg; in severe hypertension may be increased to max. 40 mg	2.5, 5, 10 and 20	Removed by dialysis	Ednyt, Enacard, Innovace, Pralenal	APS, Cox, Dexcel, Dominion, Genus, MSD, Norton, Opus, Sovereign, Sterwin
Fosinopril	11.5 (fosinoprilat)	Hydrolysed to fosinoprilat in gut and liver; excreted in urine and bile	Yes	10 mg initially, increased if necessary after 4 weeks, usual dose range 10–40 mg	10 and 20 (of fosinopril sodium)	Not removed by dialysis	Staril	Squibb

continued overleaf

Table 9.1 Contd.

ACE inhibitor	Half-life (h)	Elimination	Prodrug?	Daily dose	Tablet strength (mg)	Comments	Proprietary name(s) (UK)	Manufacturer(s) (UK)
Imidapril hydrochloride	>24 (imidaprilat)	Hydrolysed to imidaprilat; excreted in urine and faeces	Yes	5 mg initially; increase if necessary at intervals of at least 3 weeks to usual maintenance 10 mg; max. 20 mg (elderly 10 mg)	5, 10 and 20	Give before food (fat-rich meal significantly reduces absorption). Initial dose 2.5 mg in elderly, with diuretic, in heart failure, angina, cerebro-vascular disease, renal or hepatic impairment	Tanatril	Trinity
Lisinopril	12	Excreted unchanged in urine	No	2.5 mg initially; usual maintenance 10–20 mg; max. 40 mg	2.5, 5, 10 and 20	Removed by dialysis	Carace, Zestril	AstraZeneca, Du Pont

Table 9.1 Contd.

ACE inhibitor	Half-life (h)	Elimination	Prodrug?	Daily dose	Tablet strength (mg)	Comments	Proprietary name(s) (UK)	Manufacturer(s) (UK)
Moexipril hydrochloride	12 (moexiprilat)	Metabolised to moexiprilat in gut and liver; excreted mainly in urine, some in faeces	Yes	7.5 mg initially; usual range 15–30 mg	7.5 and 15	Initial dose 3.75 mg daily if taken with a diuretic, with nifedipine, in elderly, or in renal or hepatic impairment	Perdix	Schwarz
Perindopril	25–30 (perindoprilat)	Metabolised in liver to perindoprilat; excreted mainly in urine, some in faeces	Yes	2 mg initially; usual maintenance 4 mg; max. 8 mg	2 and 4 (of perindopril erbumine)	Give before food	Coversyl	Servier

continued overleaf

Table 9.1 Contd.

ACE inhibitor	Half-life (h)	Elimination	Prodrug?	Daily dose	Tablet strength (mg)	Comments	Proprietary name(s) (UK)	Manufacturer(s) (UK)
Quinapril	25 (quinaprilat)	Metabolised in liver to quinaprilat; excreted mainly in urine, some in faeces	Yes	10 mg initially; usual maintenance 20–40 mg (in single or two divided doses); up to 80 mg has been given	5, 10, 20 and 40	Initial dose 2.5 mg daily in elderly, renal impairment or taken with diuretic. Not significantly removed by dialysis	Accupro	Parke-Davis
Ramipril	13–17 (ramiprilat, following doses of 5–10 mg)	Metabolised in liver to ramiprilat; excreted in urine (60%) and faeces	Yes	1.25 mg initially increased at intervals of 1–2 weeks to usual range 2.5–5 mg; max. 10 mg	1.25, 2.5, 5 and 10	Half-life is prolonged with doses 1.25–2.5 mg daily	Tritace	Hoechst Marion Roussel

Table 9.1 Contd.

ACE inhibitor	Half-life (h)	Elimination	Prodrug?	Daily dose	Tablet strength (mg)	Comments	Proprietary name(s) (UK)	Manufacturer(s) (UK)
Trandolapril	16–24 (trandolaprilat)	Metabolised in liver to trandolaprilat; excreted in urine (33%) and faeces	Yes	0.5 mg initially, increased at intervals of 2–4 weeks to usual range 1–2 mg; max. 4 mg	0.5, 1 and 2	Not significantly removed by dialysis	Gopten, Odrik	Knoll, Hoechst Marion Roussel

Adverse effects

At one time some of the adverse effects of ACE inhibitors, such as skin reactions and taste disturbances, were thought to be due to the presence of the sulfhydryl group, as in captopril. Now, though, it is considered that all ACE inhibitors share a similar range of adverse effects, most of which are reversible on stopping treatment.[5,6]

Hypotension

The first few doses of an ACE inhibitor can produce pronounced hypotension. The drop in blood pressure can be severe enough to provoke a myocardial infarction or cerebrovascular accident in those with ischaemic heart disease or cerebrovascular disease. Certain patients are especially at risk of hypotension, for example, patients with heart failure and sodium- or volume-depleted patients. To minimise problems with hypotension, the first dose of an ACE inhibitor should preferably be given at bedtime. In those patients particularly likely to suffer hypotension (see above and Adverse Effects Focus, p. 89), treatment should be started under close medical supervision, using a low dose, and with the patient in a recumbent position. Symptomatic hypotension generally responds to lying the patient down and volume expansion either with oral fluids or with an intravenous infusion of sodium chloride 0.9%. Specific therapy with angiotensin amide may be considered if these measures are ineffective.

Renal effects

ACE inhibitors can cause increases in blood concentrations of urea and creatinine.[2,7] Proteinuria may also occur. Some patients have gone on to develop reversible acute renal failure and nephrotic syndrome. These effects occur mainly in those who already have renal or renovascular dysfunction. Patients with heart failure are also more susceptible and hypovolaemia may be an aggravating factor. The deterioration in renal function can sometimes be dramatic; patients with bilateral renal artery stenosis are particularly at risk. Serum urea and creatinine must be checked before and a few weeks after starting an ACE inhibitor.

Cough

A persistent, non-productive cough is a common adverse effect of ACE inhibitors.[8-10] It may occur soon after the ACE inhibitor is started or may not appear until after weeks or even months of treatment. The cough may be accompanied by voice changes (hoarseness or huskiness) and is often worse when lying down. Women, non-smokers and older patients seem to be especially susceptible. The cough is a result of increased sensitivity of the cough reflex, although what produces this is not certain; locally produced prostaglandins or bradykinin or substance P (both substrates for ACE) have been suggested.

Although spontaneous recovery or improvement in the cough has been reported, in most cases the cough persists. Sometimes reducing the dose may help and various drugs have been tried, including non-steroidal anti-inflammatory drugs (NSAIDs), nifedipine, inhaled bupivacaine, inhaled sodium cromoglicate, oral baclofen and oral picotamide. Changing to an alternative ACE inhibitor is not advised since it is rarely effective. In many patients, though, there is no alternative but to withdraw the ACE inhibitor.

Effects on electrolytes

The ACE inhibitors can cause hyperkalaemia because they reduce aldosterone and thus potassium excretion. They also produce hyponatraemia.

Effects on the blood

Blood disorders, including neutropenia and agranulocytosis, may occur, especially in patients with renal failure and in those with collagen vascular disorders such as systemic lupus erythematosus and scleroderma. Thrombocytopenia and anaemias have also been reported.

Angioedema

Angioedema is a rare side-effect, occurring in about 0.1–0.2% of patients. It can affect the face, lips, tongue, glottis, larynx and extremities and occurs especially in the first few weeks, although it can occur at any time. Patients should be warned that medical attention should be sought for signs of facial or extremity swelling or if they have difficulty in swallowing or breathing. The ACE inhibitor should be withdrawn immediately. Antihistamines may be needed in some cases and if the swelling is likely to result in obstruction of the airway, subcutaneous adrenaline (epinephrine) should be given.

Other side-effects

Other side-effects include chest pain, palpitations, tachycardia, alopecia, stomatitis, dizziness, fatigue, headache, gastrointestinal disturbances, taste disturbances, abdominal pain, pancreatitis, hepatocellular injury or cholestatic jaundice, muscle cramps, paraesthesias, mood and sleep disturbances and impotence. Rarer side-effects include skin rashes (including erythema multiforme and toxic epidermal necrolysis) and a symptom complex that includes fever and vasculitis. Upper respiratory tract symptoms and hypersensitivity reactions have also been reported.

Drug interactions[11-13]

The antihypertensive effect of ACE inhibitors is enhanced by concomitant administration with other drugs that have a secondary hypotensive effect. In some cases excessive hypotension may occur; this is also a risk when ACE inhibitors are given with diuretics or other antihypertensive drugs. The antihypertensive effect of ACE inhibitors may be antagonised by administration with other drugs that have a hypertensive effect (see Chapter 16).

Blood adverse effects enhanced

There is an increased risk of neutropenia or agranulocytosis (especially in patients with renal impairment) if ACE inhibitors are given together with immunosuppressants, allopurinol or procainamide.

Hyperkalaemic effect enhanced

Serum potassium concentrations must be monitored if an ACE inhibitor is used in combination with potassium-sparing diuretics, potassium supplements (including potassium-containing salt substitutes) or other drugs that can cause hyperkalaemia, such as ciclosporin or indometacin. Patients with heart failure who are taking potassium-sparing diuretics and potassium supplements must stop taking these before they start treatment with an ACE inhibitor.

Renal adverse effects enhanced

Other drugs, such as NSAIDs and ciclosporin, which can affect renal function, may potentiate the adverse effects of ACE inhibitors on the kidneys.

Allopurinol

Fatal Stevens–Johnson syndrome and a hypersensitivity reaction (fever, arthralgia, myalgia) have been reported in two patients with chronic renal failure when allopurinol was added to established treatment with captopril. See also above for effects on blood.

Antacids

Antacids can reduce the absorption of captopril, fosinopril and possibly other ACE inhibitors administered concurrently.

Antidiabetics

Hypoglycaemia has been reported following introduction of ACE inhibitor therapy both in diabetic patients on insulin or oral hypoglycaemics and in non-diabetic patients. This effect has been attributed to enhanced insulin sensitivity. However, other studies have failed to find any effect on blood sugar levels and ACE inhibitors have been favoured by some as first-line drugs in the treatment of hypertension in diabetic patients. Patients should be warned that hypoglycaemia could occur and it is suggested that the dose of hypoglycaemic should be reduced when the ACE inhibitor is started.

Ciclosporin

Ciclosporin can have an additive hyperkalaemic effect with ACE inhibitors (see p. 98). The combination of ciclosporin with an ACE inhibitor may also cause additive renal toxicity; acute renal failure that resolved once the ACE inhibitor was withdrawn has been reported in two patients receiving ciclosporin after renal transplantation.

Digoxin

Although there have been some reports of increased serum digoxin concentrations in some patients with heart failure also taking an ACE inhibitor, other studies have failed to find any interaction. However, since ACE inhibitors can reduce renal function that would reduce the excretion of digoxin, the combination should be used with caution.

General anaesthetics

Marked hypotension may occur in patients on ACE inhibitors when they undergo general anaesthesia. It has also been reported that corrected cerebral blood flow was significantly lower in patients who were taking captopril before general anaesthesia compared with patients pretreated with metoprolol and untreated controls and it has been suggested that discontinuation of ACE inhibitor therapy before anaesthesia should be considered.

Lithium

Increased serum lithium concentrations have been reported in patients also taking an ACE inhibitor, possibly due to ACE inhibitor effects on reducing glomerular filtration and concentration of sodium in the proximal tubule.

NSAIDs

NSAIDs may interact with ACE inhibitors in a number of ways and the combination should be used with caution. Antagonism of the antihypertensive effect of ACE inhibitors by NSAIDs is discussed in Chapter 16. Indometacin and possibly other NSAIDs may have an additive hyperkalaemic effect with ACE inhibitors.

Of more concern is the possibility of an interaction between low-dose aspirin and ACE inhibitors, especially in patients with heart failure. In a study in patients with severe heart failure aspirin appeared to counteract the vasodilator activity of enalapril.[14] The clinical implications for patients with less severe left ventricular dysfunction are not clear and review of the evidence for such an interaction has concluded that the data were inconclusive and further study was required.[15]

Since NSAIDs and ACE inhibitors act at different parts of the glomerulus, the combination may have variable effects on renal function. The combination can cause deterioration in renal function when given to patients whose kidneys are underperfused (for example, in heart failure, liver cirrhosis or haemorrhage), although in patients with normal renal perfusion the combination may produce some benefit.

Preparations

See Table 9.1.

References

1. Schachter M, ed. *ACE Inhibitors; Current Use and Future Prospects*. London: Martin Dunitz, 1995.
2. Navis G, Faber H J, de Zeeuw D, de Jong P E. ACE inhibitors and the kidney: a risk–benefit assessment. *Drug Safety* 1996; 15: 200–211.
3. Burnier M, Biollaz J. Pharmacokinetic optimisation of angiotensin converting enzyme (ACE) inhibitor therapy. *Clin Pharmacokinet* 1992; 22: 375–384.
4. Hoyer J, Schulte K J, Lenz T. Clinical pharmacokinetics of angiotensin converting enzyme (ACE) inhibitors in renal failure. *Clin Pharmacokinet* 1993; 24: 230–254.
5. Parish R C, Miller L J. Adverse effects of angiotensin converting enzyme (ACE) inhibitors: an update. *Drug Safety* 1992; 7: 14–31.
6. Alderman C P. Adverse effects of the angiotensin-converting enzyme inhibitors. *Ann Pharmacother* 1996; 30: 55–61.
7. Gans R O B, Hoorntje S J, Donker A J. Renal effects of angiotensin-I converting enzyme inhibitors. *Neth J Med* 1988; 32: 247–264.
8. Anonymous. Cough caused by ACE inhibitors. *Drug Ther Bull* 1994; 32: 28, 55–56.
9. Ravid D, Lishner M, Lang R, Ravid M. Angiotensin-converting enzyme inhibitors and cough: a prospective evaluation in hypertension and congestive heart failure. *J Clin Pharmacol* 1994; 34: 1116–1120.
10. Overlack A. ACE inhibitor-induced cough and bronchospasm. *Drug Safety* 1996; 15: 72–78.
11. Shionoiri H. Pharmacokinetic drug interactions with ACE inhibitors. *Clin Pharmacokinet* 1993; 25: 20–58.
12. Mignat C, Unger T. ACE inhibitors: drug interactions of clinical significance. *Drug Safety* 1995; 12: 334–337.
13. Stockley I H. *Drug Interactions*, 5th edn. London: Pharmaceutical Press, 1999.
14. Hall D, Zeitler H, Rudolph W. Counteraction of the vasodilator effects of enalapril by aspirin in severe heart failure. *J Am Coll Cardiol* 1992; 20: 1549–1555.
15. Cleland J G F, Bulpitt C J, Falk R H, *et al*. Is aspirin safe for patients with heart failure? *Br Heart J* 1995; 74: 215–219.

10

Calcium-channel blockers

Indications

Calcium-channel blockers are alternative first-line antihypertensives that may be considered in patients who have contraindications to or who do not tolerate thiazide diuretics or beta blockers. They are particularly indicated in patients who have angina and in elderly patients with isolated systolic hypertension. They may be used as sole therapy or may be combined with an angiotensin-converting enzyme (ACE) inhibitor. Dihydropyridine calcium-channel blockers and possibly diltiazem may also be used in combination with a beta blocker.

Mechanism of action[1]

Verapamil was the first of the calcium-channel blockers to be introduced into clinical practice, originally for angina pectoris, in 1970. Since then many different calcium-channel blockers have been developed with a wide range of clinical uses.

Calcium-channel blockers, also known as calcium antagonists, calcium-entry blockers and slow-channel blockers, act by interfering with the inward displacement of calcium ions through the slow channels in the cell membrane that is responsible for maintenance of the plateau phase of the action potential. The main tissues affected by calcium-channel blockers are therefore those in which depolarisation is dependent on calcium influx rather than sodium influx. Such tissues include vascular smooth muscle, myocardial cells and cells within the sinoatrial and atrioventricular nodes. Blockade of calcium channels in these tissues produces the following effects: dilatation of coronary and peripheral arteries and arterioles (with little or no effect on venous tone); a negative inotropic action; a reduction in heart rate; and a slowing of atrioventricular conduction.

However, the calcium-channel blockers differ in their selectivity for the various different tissues and therefore individual calcium-channel blockers may not produce all these effects and thus have different clinical uses. The various calcium-channel blockers available may be classified according to their chemical structure into three major groups: dihydropyridine-type (nifedipine), benzothiazepine (diltiazem) and phenylalkylamine (verapamil) calcium-channel blockers (see Figure 10.1). These structural differences correlate largely with differences in selectivity and these are outlined below.

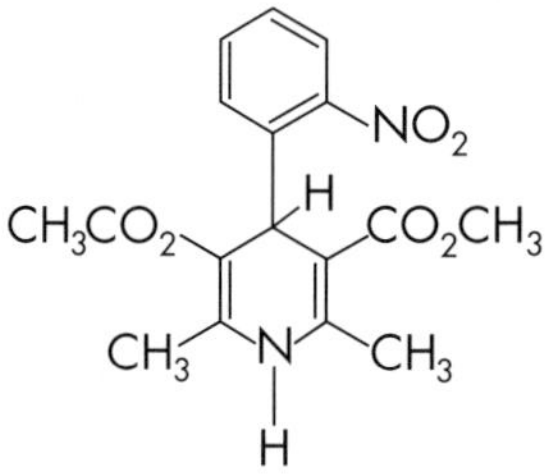

Nifedipine

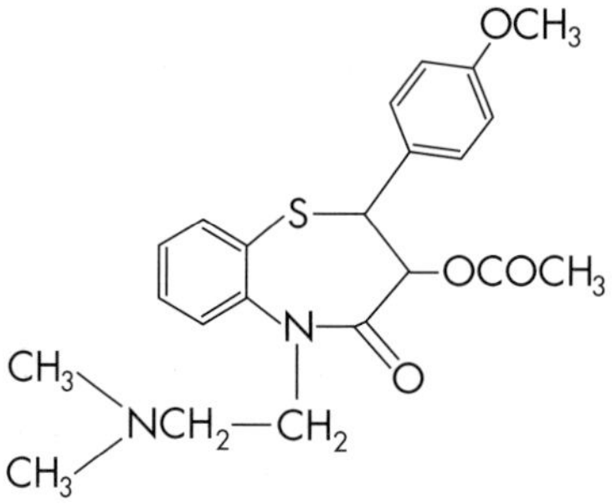

Diltiazem

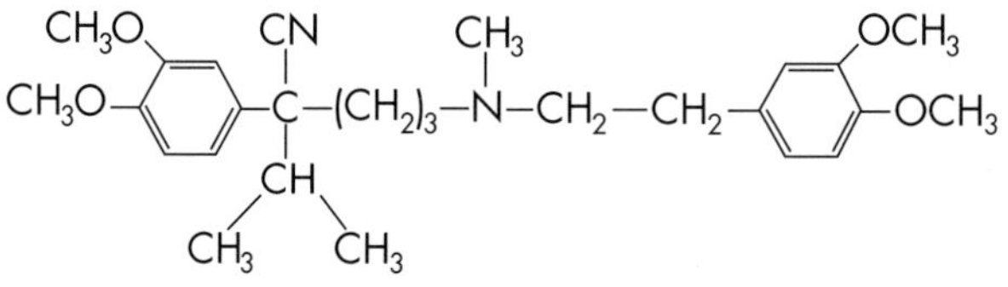

Verapamil

Figure 10.1 Calcium-channel blockers.

Dihydropyridine-type

Dihydropyridine calcium-channel blockers, such as nifedipine and amlodipine, have a greater selectivity for calcium channels in vascular smooth muscle than for those in myocardium and therefore their main effect is vasodilatation of both coronary and peripheral arteries producing reduced peripheral resistance and blood pressure. There is a reflex increase in heart rate. They have little or no action at the sinoatrial or atrioventricular nodes and negative inotropic activity is rarely seen at therapeutic doses. Nicardipine and newer dihydropyridines such as amlodipine, felodipine, isradipine and lacidipine may be even more selective than nifedipine for vascular smooth muscle. Most of the dihydropyridine calcium-channel blockers (nifedipine and lacidipine are exceptions) are chiral compounds used as racemic mixtures.

Diltiazem

Diltiazem is a benzothiazepine calcium-channel blocker that has peripheral and coronary vasodilator properties, although its vasodilator properties are less marked than those of the dihydropyridine calcium-channel blockers. Diltiazem also inhibits cardiac conduction, particularly at the sinoatrial and atrioventricular nodes, but it has less negative inotropic effect than verapamil and significant myocardial depression occurs rarely.

Verapamil

Verapamil is a much less selective vasodilator than the dihydropyridine calcium-channel blockers and is highly negatively inotropic. It acts as an antihypertensive by its effects of reducing peripheral vascular resistance, but it also acts on myocardium, causing depression of sinoatrial and atrioventricular nodal conduction, and thus slows the heart rate. Verapamil also reduces coronary vascular resistance.

Pharmacokinetics[1,2]

Dihydropyridine-type

Dihydropyridine calcium-channel blockers are well-absorbed after oral administration, with the exception of lacidipine. However, they undergo extensive first-pass metabolism. All are highly bound to plasma proteins.

They are extensively metabolised in the liver and are excreted largely as metabolites either mainly in the urine (amlodipine, nifedipine) or in the urine and faeces (felodipine, isradipine, lacidipine, lercanidipine, nicardipine, nisoldipine).

Diltiazem

Diltiazem undergoes rapid and almost complete absorption from the gastrointestinal tract after oral administration. However, there is extensive first-pass hepatic metabolism and bioavailability has been reported to be about 40%. There is considerable interindividual variation in plasma concentrations. Diltiazem is about 80% bound to plasma proteins and is widely distributed. It undergoes extensive metabolism in the liver and one of the metabolites formed, desacetyldiltiazem, has been reported to have 25–50% of the activity of the parent compound. Diltiazem is excreted largely as metabolites in bile and urine. It is poorly dialysable.

Verapamil[3]

Verapamil is well absorbed after oral administration, but is subject to considerable first-pass metabolism in the liver and the bioavailability is only about 20%. There is considerable interindividual variation in plasma verapamil concentrations. Verapamil is widely distributed. It is about 90% bound to plasma proteins. Verapamil is extensively metabolised in the liver to at least 12 metabolites; one metabolite, norverapamil, has been shown to have some activity. The majority of a dose is excreted by the kidneys as metabolites; about 16% is excreted in the bile. Verapamil is not removed by dialysis.

Dosage

See Table 10.1. Many of the calcium-channel blockers are available in normal-release and modified-release formulations; the dose usually depends on the formulation used. Short-acting preparations of nifedipine are not recommended for the management of hypertension. Diltiazem is available in standard and long-acting formulations (although they are all designated modified-release). Some of the long-acting preparations are given twice a day and some once a day and therefore patients should be prescribed these formulations by brand name.

Table 10.1 Calcium-channel blockers

Calcium-channel blocker	Type	Half-life (h)	Elimination	Daily dose	Tablet strength (mg)	Comments	Proprietary name(s) (UK)	Manufacturer(s) (UK)
Amlodipine besilate	Dihydropyridine	35–50	Metabolised in liver; excreted mostly in urine	5 mg initially; max. 10 mg	5 and 10 (of amlodipine)		Istin	Pfizer
Diltiazem hydrochloride	Benzothiazepine	3–5	Metabolised in liver; excreted in urine and bile	Dose depends on formulation	60, 90, 120, 180, 200, 240, 300 and 360	Reduce dose in hepatic and renal impairment	Adizem-SR, Adizem-XL, Angiozem, Angitil SR, Angitil XL, Calcicard CR, Dilcardia SR, Dilzem SR, Dilzem XL, Optil, Slozem, Tildiem, Tildiem LA, Tildiem Retard, Viazem XL, Zemtard	Ashbourne, Cox, Du Pont, Elan, Galen, Generics, Hill cross, Lipha, Napp, Norton, Opus, Sanofi-Synthelabo, Sterwin, Trinity

continued overleaf

Table 10.1 Contd.

Calcium-channel blocker	Type	Half-life (h)	Elimination	Daily dose	Tablet strength (mg)	Comments	Proprietary name(s) (UK)	Manufacturer(s) (UK)
Felodipine	Dihydropyridine	11–16	Metabolised in gut and liver; excreted in urine (70%) and bile	5 mg initially (elderly 2.5 mg); usual maintenance 5–10 mg, doses above 20 mg rarely needed	2.5, 5 and 10	Should be taken in the morning. Reduced doses may be needed in liver impairment	Plendil	AstraZeneca
Isradipine	Dihydropyridine	8 (some studies report less than 4 h)	Metabolised in liver; excreted in urine (65%) and bile	5 mg initially (elderly, hepatic or renal impairment 2.5 mg), increased if necessary after 3–4 weeks to 10 mg (exceptionally 20 mg)	2.5	Daily doses given in two divided doses. Maintenance dose of 2.5 or 5 mg daily (not divided) may be sufficient	Prescal	Novartis

Table 10.1 Contd.

Calcium-channel blocker	Type	Half-life (h)	Elimination	Daily dose	Tablet strength (mg)	Comments	Proprietary name(s) (UK)	Manufacturer(s) (UK)
Lacidipine	Dihydropyridine	13–19	Metabolised in liver; excreted in bile (70%) and urine	2 mg initially, increased after 3–4 weeks to 4 mg; max. 6 mg	2 and 4	Give preferably in the morning	Motens	Boehringer Ingelheim
Lercanidipine hydrochloride	Dihydropyridine	2–5	Metabolised in liver; 50% excreted in urine	10 mg initially, increased if necessary after at least 2 weeks to 20 mg	10		Zanidip	Napp
Nicardipine hydrochloride	Dihydropyridine	8	Metabolised in liver; excreted in urine and bile	60 mg initially (in three divided doses), increased after at least 3 days to 90 mg (usual range 60–120 mg)	20 and 30	Non-linear pharma-cokinetics due to saturable first-pass metabolism. A modified-release preparation also available. Reduced doses may be needed in liver impairment	Cardene	Yamanouchi

continued overleaf

Table 10.1 Contd.

Calcium-channel blocker	Type	Half-life (h)	Elimination	Daily dose	Tablet strength (mg)	Comments	Proprietary name(s) (UK)	Manufacturer(s) (UK)
Nifedipine	Dihydropyridine	Half-life depends on dosage form; 6–11 (tablets), 2–3.4 (capsules)	Metabolised in liver; excreted in urine	Dose depends on formulation	10, 20, 30, 40 and 60	Liquid-filled capsules are available but are not recommended for use in hypertension. Reduced doses may be needed in liver impairment	Adalat LA, Adalat Retard, Adipine MR, Angiopine 40 LA, Angiopine MR, Cardilate MR, Coracten SR, Coracten XL, Coroday MR, Fortipine LA 40, Hypolar Retard 20, Nifedipress MR, Nifedotard 20 MR, Nifopress Retard, Nimodrel MR, Slofedipine, Slofedipine XL, Tensipine MR	Ashbourne, Bayer, Cox, Dexcel, Galen, Generics, Genus, Gold shield, Lagap, Medeva, Norton, Opus, Sterwin, Trinity

Table 10.1 Contd.

Calcium-channel blocker	Type	Half-life (h)	Elimination	Daily dose	Tablet strength (mg)	Comments	Proprietary name(s) (UK)	Manufacturer(s) (UK)
Nisoldipine	Dihydropyridine	7–12	Metabolised in gut and liver; excreted in urine (60–80%) and bile	10 mg initially, increased if necessary at intervals of at least 1 week to max. 40 mg	10, 20 and 30	Give preferably before breakfast	Syscor MR	Pharmax
Verapamil hydrochloride	Phenylalkylamine	4.5–12 (with repeated doses)	Metabolised in liver; excreted in urine (70%) and bile	Dose depends on formulation	40, 80, 120, 160, 180 and 240	Reduce dose in liver impairment	Cordilox, Cordilox MR, Ethimil MR, Half Securon SR, Securon, Securon SR, Univer, Verapress MR, Vertab SR 240	APS, Baker Norton, Cox, Dexcel, Elan, Genus, Hill-cross, Knoll, Norton, Trinity

Adverse effects[4]

Effects on the heart

Verapamil's effects on cardiac conduction can produce various adverse effects including bradycardia, atrioventricular block, worsening heart failure and transient asystole. These effects may be particularly severe in patients with hypertrophic cardiomyopathy and are more common with parenteral than with oral therapy. These effects on conduction mean that verapamil is contraindicated or must be used with caution in those with conduction disorders or heart failure (see Adverse Effects Focus, below) and should not be used with other drugs affecting cardiac conduction (see p. 114).

ADVERSE EFFECTS FOCUS

Contraindications and cautions for calcium-channel blockers

- Hypotension – verapamil contraindicated, dihydropyridine-type caution
- Cardiogenic shock – verapamil and dihydropyridine-type contraindicated
- Marked bradycardia – verapamil and diltiazem contraindicated
- Atrioventricular block – verapamil and diltiazem contraindicated in second- or third-degree block, caution in lesser degrees of block
- Heart failure or impaired left ventricular function – verapamil contraindicated, diltiazem should usually be avoided, caution with dihydropyridine-type
- Sick-sinus syndrome – verapamil and diltiazem contraindicated
- Severe aortic stenosis – dihydropyridine-type contraindicated (increased risk of developing heart failure)
- Unstable angina – dihydropyridine-type contraindicated
- Sudden withdrawal of calcium-channel blockers may be associated with an exacerbation of angina
- Wolff–Parkinson–White syndrome complicated by atrial flutter or fibrillation – verapamil usually contraindicated (may induce severe ventricular tachycardia)

Diltiazem can similarly cause conduction problems, although less frequently than verapamil, and similar cautions apply.

Dihydropyridine-type calcium-channel blockers have little or no effect on cardiac conduction at therapeutic doses, although there are rare reports of heart block, and they are best avoided in patients with heart failure. Short-acting formulations of nifedipine are not recommended for angina or long-term management of hypertension; their use may be associated with large variations in blood pressure and reflex tachycardia that can provoke or aggravate ischaemic chest pain. This is especially likely just after starting therapy. In a few patients excessive fall in blood pressure has led to cerebral or myocardial ischaemia or transient blindness. Dihydropyridine-type calcium-channel blockers should be discontinued in patients who experience ischaemic pain following its administration.

Gastrointestinal effects

The most troublesome non-cardiac side-effect occurring with verapamil is constipation, as a result of reduced intestinal motility. Nausea may also occur but is less frequently reported. Diltiazem can cause gastrointestinal problems that include anorexia, vomiting, constipation or diarrhoea, taste disturbances and weight gain; these occur less frequently than the gastrointestinal problems seen with verapamil. Nausea and other gastrointestinal disturbances have occurred with dihydropyridine-type calcium-channel blockers.

Hypersensitivity reactions

Hypersensitivity reactions, including skin reactions and transient elevations in liver enzyme values, have occurred with calcium-channel blockers. The skin reactions (erythema and urticaria) are usually mild and transient, although a few cases of erythema multiforme and exfoliative dermatitis have occurred.[5] Hepatitis has been reported occasionally.

Increased mortality

For a discussion of the controversy over possible increased mortality with calcium-channel blockers (especially short-acting nifedipine and high doses), see p. 35.

Vasodilatory effects

The most common problems with the dihydropyridine calcium-channel blockers are vasodilatory effects such as palpitations, tachycardia, headaches, flushing, hypotension and peripheral oedema of the feet and ankles. These effects often diminish on continued therapy. The peripheral oedema occurs typically 2 weeks or more after starting therapy and if it does not diminish on continued therapy might respond to simple measures such as elevation of the feet or a reduction in dosage. Combination with a beta blocker helps to reduce these symptoms but does not eliminate this problem. Vasodilatory effects may also occur with diltiazem and verapamil.

Other side-effects

Gingival hyperplasia that resolves on drug withdrawal has been reported with calcium-channel blockers.[6] Fatigue may occur. Gynaecomastia has been reported with some calcium-channel blockers. Increased micturition frequency, lethargy, eye pain and mental depression have occurred with dihydropyridine-type calcium-channel blockers. Hyperglycaemia has been observed with dihydropyridine calcium-channel blockers (see below).

Drug interactions[7,8]

The antihypertensive effect of calcium-channel blockers is enhanced by concomitant administration with other drugs that have a secondary hypotensive effect and antagonised by administration with other drugs that have a hypertensive effect (see Chapter 16).

Antidiabetics

Nifedipine may modify insulin and glucose responses and therefore diabetic patients may need to adjust their antidiabetic treatment when receiving nifedipine.

Beta blockers

Verapamil should not be used in conjunction with a beta blocker due to the additive cardiodepressant effect. The combination of intravenous verapamil with a beta blocker is especially hazardous. Diltiazem is also best avoided in conjunction with a beta blocker, although some authorities say the combination may be used with caution. A dihydropyridine calcium-channel blocker is often used with a beta blocker without untoward effects, although heart failure and severe hypotension have been reported in a few patients.

Cardiac depressants

Verapamil and diltiazem should be avoided or used with extreme caution in combination with other drugs that have myocardial depressant effects, such as antiarrhythmics, mefloquine, digoxin, some general anaesthetics or drugs with beta blocking effects (see also Beta blockers, above). The increased depression of cardiac conduction increases the risk of bradycardia and atrioventricular block.

Enzyme inducers and inhibitors

Calcium-channel blockers are metabolised in the liver by the cytochrome P450 enzyme system and interactions may occur with other drugs that are subject to hepatic oxidation. Interactions may also occur with enzyme inducers, such as carbamazepine, phenobarbital, phenytoin and rifampicin, and enzyme inhibitors, such as azole antifungals, cimetidine and erythromycin. Grapefruit juice contains an inhibitor of the cytochrome P450 enzyme system that particularly affects enzyme in the intestinal wall. It should not be consumed at the same time as oral dihydropyridine calcium-channel blockers or verapamil. Nifedipine is metabolised by the same pathway as quinidine; there are some reports of increased nifedipine serum concentrations and some of reduced plasma quinidine concentrations. Diltiazem and verapamil can themselves inhibit the metabolism of other drugs that are subject to metabolism by cytochrome P450; increased plasma concentrations of many drugs, including carbamazepine, ciclosporin, midazolam and theophylline, may occur. The plasma concentrations of alcohol and digoxin may also be increased.

Lithium

Combination of verapamil with lithium may increase sensitivity to lithium and enhance neurotoxicity. Neurotoxicity has also been reported in patients taking diltiazem and lithium.

Preparations

See Table 10.1.

References

1.   Epstein M, ed. *Calcium Antagonists in Clinical Medicine*, 2nd edn. Philadelphia: Hanley & Belfus, 1997.

2.   Kelly J G, O'Malley K. Clinical pharmacokinetics of calcium antagonists: an update. *Clin Pharmacokinet* 1992; 22: 416–433.
3.   Hamann S R, Blouin R A, McAllister R G. Clinical pharmacokinetics of verapamil. *Clin Pharmacokinet* 1984; 9: 26–41.
4.   Dougall H T, McLay J. A comparative review of the adverse effects of calcium antagonists. *Drug Safety* 1996; 15: 91–106.
5.   Stern R, Khalsa J H. Cutaneous adverse reactions associated with calcium channel blockers. *Arch Intern Med* 1989; 149: 829–832.
6.   Steele R M, Schuna A A, Schreiber R T. Calcium antagonist-induced gingival hyperplasia. *Ann Intern Med* 1994; 120: 663–664.
7.   Stockley I H. *Drug Interactions*, 5th edn. London: Pharmaceutical Press, 1999.
8.   Rosenthal T, Ezra D. Calcium antagonists: drug interactions of clinical significance. *Drug Safety* 1995; 13: 157–187.

11

Alpha blockers

Indications

The alpha blockers are alternative first-choice agents that may be used when there are contraindications to beta blockers or thiazides. They are particularly indicated in patients who also have benign prostatic hyperplasia. They can be used in combination with any of the other major antihypertensive drugs. They are not associated with adverse changes in serum lipid profile or effects on glucose and may therefore be useful in patients with dyslipidaemia or glucose intolerance.

Mechanism of action

Alpha blockers are also known as alpha-adrenergic antagonists or alpha-adrenergic receptor antagonists. Alpha blockers produce vasodilatation by blocking the action of noradrenaline (norepinephrine) at post-synaptic alpha$_1$ adrenoceptors in both arterioles and veins. This results in a fall in peripheral resistance and thus blood pressure. There is usually little compensatory rise in cardiac output (reflex tachycardia). They reduce both standing and supine blood pressure, with a greater effect on diastolic pressure. The alpha blockers covered in this chapter (doxazosin, prazosin, terazosin and indoramin: see Figure 11.1) are all competitive inhibitors that act selectively at the alpha$_1$ adrenoceptor. The older alpha blockers, phentolamine and phenoxybenzamine, have been available for several decades and are non-selective alpha blockers, that is, they act at both alpha$_1$ and alpha$_2$ adrenoceptors. They are used mainly in the management of phaeochromocytoma. They have been used rarely in the general treatment of hypertension because of the high incidence of adverse effects that are due to catecholamine release (tachycardia and tolerance). The newer selective alpha blockers are not associated with these adverse effects.

Alpha blockers also act at alpha adrenoceptors in non-vascular smooth muscle, for example in the bladder, where alpha blockade produces decreased resistance to urinary outflow. This property

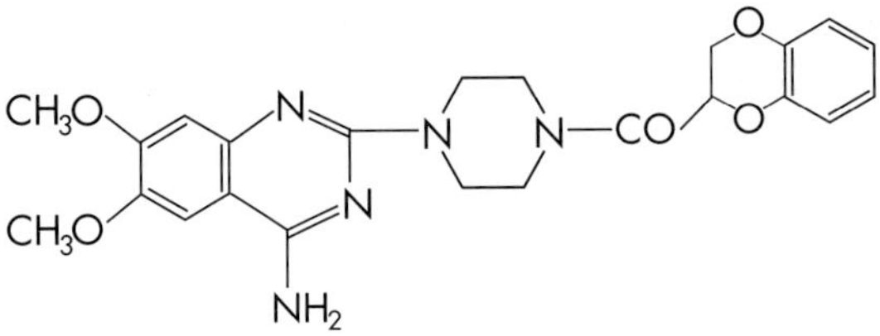

Doxazosin

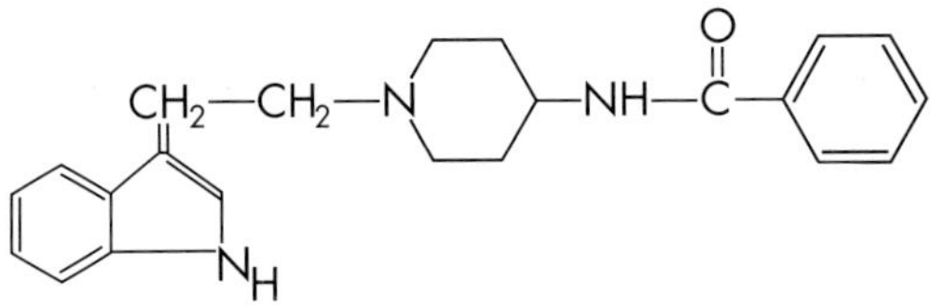

Indoramin

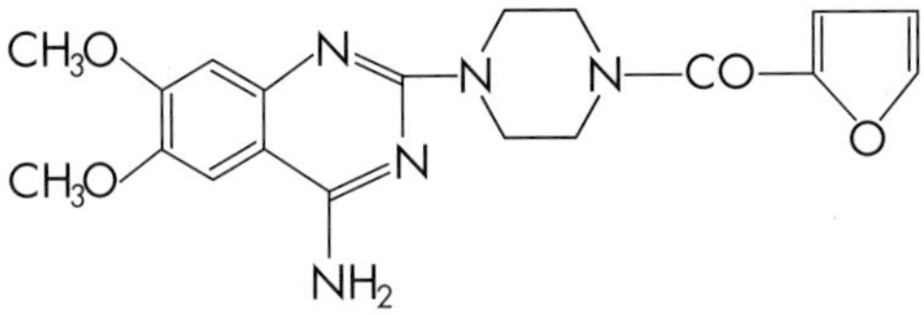

Prazosin

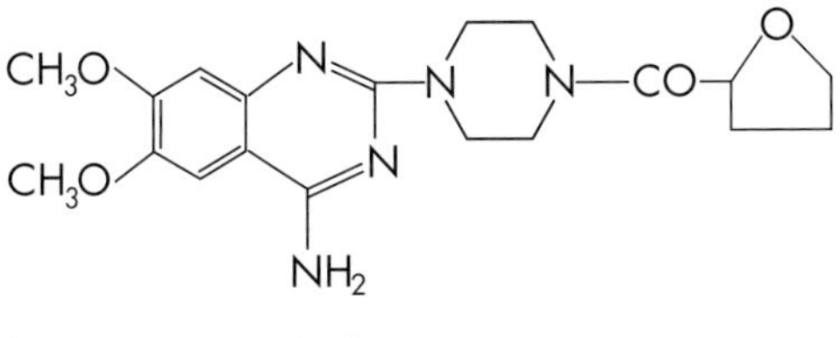

Terazosin

Figure 11.1 Alpha blockers.

makes alpha blockers useful in the treatment of benign prostatic hypertrophy.

Prazosin was the first of the selective alpha blockers to be developed. It is short-acting and tends to produce precipitous falls in blood pressure. Doxazosin and terazosin are longer-acting and therefore produce a more gentle reduction in blood pressure and may be given once daily. Indoramin, in addition to its alpha blocking activity, possesses membrane-stabilising properties and is a competitive antagonist at histamine H_1 and 5-hydroxytryptamine receptors.

In contrast to beta blockers and thiazide diuretics, alpha blockers actually produce modest improvements in serum lipids (reduction in total cholesterol and low-density lipoprotein (LDL)-cholesterol)[1] and glucose tolerance, although whether this translates into improved outcomes is not known.

Contraindications

Doxazosin, prazosin and terazosin should be used with caution in patients with angina pectoris. Indoramin should be avoided in patients with heart failure and caution is necessary if it is used in patients with depression or a history of epilepsy.

Pharmacokinetics[2]

Alpha bockers are well absorbed after oral administration but they vary considerably in their bioavailability. They all undergo metabolism in the liver; some metabolites of indoramin, prazosin and terazosin may retain some antihypertensive activity. Excretion varies slightly between alpha blockers (see Table 11.1); doxazosin is excreted exclusively in the bile, prazosin is excreted predominantly in the bile with the remainder in urine and indoramin and terazosin are excreted in bile and urine.

The alpha blockers are all highly bound to plasma proteins and are therefore unlikely to be removed by dialysis.

Dosage

See Table 11.1.

To avoid the risk of collapse which may occur in some patients after the first dose of an alpha blocker (except indoramin), the initial dose is given preferably at bedtime.

Adverse effects

Alpha blockers are, on the whole, well tolerated.[3]

Doxazosin, prazosin and terazosin

Postural hypotension

Postural hypotension, that may be severe and produce syncope following the initial dose, is the main side-effect of these alpha blockers. It may

Table 11.1 Alpha blockers

Alpha blocker	Half-life (h)	Elimination	Daily dose	Tablet strength (mg)	Comments	Proprietary name(s) (UK)	Manufacturer(s) (UK)
Doxazosin	22	Extensively metabolised; excreted mainly in faeces	1 mg, increased after 1–2 weeks to 2 mg and thereafter to 4 mg, if necessary; max. 16 mg	1 (as mesilate)		Cardura	Invicta
Indoramin	5	Extensively metabolised; excreted in urine (35%) and faeces (46%)	50 mg initially (in two divided doses), increased by 25–50 mg daily at intervals of 2 weeks; max. 200 mg (in 2–3 divided doses)	25 and 50 (as hydrochloride)	Also has membrane-stabilising properties and is a competitive antagonist at H_1 and 5-hydroxy-tryptamine receptors. Lower doses may be needed in elderly	Baratol	Shire

Table 11.1 Contd.

Alpha blocker	Half-life (h)	Elimination	Daily dose	Tablet strength (mg)	Comments	Proprietary name(s) (UK)	Manufacturer(s) (UK)
Prazosin	2–4	Extensively metabolised; excreted mainly in faeces	1–1.5 mg, increased to 2–3 mg after 3–7 days; further increased if necessary to max. 20 mg	0.5, 1, 2 and 5 (as hydrochloride)	Give daily dose in 2–3 divided doses. Doses may need to be reduced in the elderly, or in renal or hepatic impairment	Alphavase, Hypovase	APS, Ashbourne, Cox, Hillcross, Invicta, Norton
Terazosin	12	Metabolised; excreted in urine (40%) and faeces (60%)	1 mg at bedtime, dose doubled after 7 days if necessary; usual maintenance 2–10 mg	2, 5 and 10 (as hydrochloride)	More than 20 mg daily rarely improves efficacy	Hytrin	Abbott

be preceded by tachycardia. To avoid this reaction treatment must be introduced cautiously, starting with a low dose, preferably at night. Doses should be increased gradually. In most patients this severe hypotension does not recur after the initial period or during subsequent titration steps. Patients should be warned to avoid standing up quickly from a lying or sitting position. Should symptoms of postural hypotension develop (dizziness, light-headedness and fainting), patients should lie down and then sit down for a few minutes before standing up to prevent their recurrence. Certain patients may be more prone to developing postural hypotension, including the elderly, patients who are volume-depleted or sodium-restricted, patients with renal or hepatic impairment, and those taking other antihypertensive therapy.

Other side-effects

The more common side-effects include dizziness, drowsiness, headache, lack of energy, nausea and palpitations. These effects may diminish on continued alpha blocker treatment or with a reduced dose. Patients affected by drowsiness or dizziness should not drive or operate machinery.

Other adverse effects include oedema, chest pain, dyspnoea, depression and nervousness, sleep disturbances, vertigo, hallucinations, transient loss of consciousness, paraesthesia, reddened sclera, blurred vision, tinnitus, abnormal liver enzyme values, pancreatitis and arthralgia. Skin disorders include rashes, pruritus and diaphoresis. Gastrointestinal effects include constipation, diarrhoea and vomiting. Upper respiratory tract disorders include nasal congestion, epistaxis and dryness of mouth. Impotence and priapism have also been reported. Alpha blockers may cause urinary incontinence,[4] particularly in women. Urinary frequency may also occur.

Indoramin

The most common adverse effects in patients receiving indoramin are sedation and dizziness and therefore care should be taken in patients who drive or operate machinery (see also Interactions below, for a warning about combination with alcohol). In common with the other alpha blockers, indoramin may cause dry mouth, nasal congestion, headache, fatigue and depression. Weight gain and failure of ejaculation may also occur. Extrapyramidal disturbances have been reported and therefore caution should be observed in using indoramin in patients with Parkinson's disease.

Drug interactions[5]

The antihypertensive effect of alpha blockers is enhanced by concomitant administration with other drugs that have a secondary hypotensive effect and antagonised by administration with other drugs that have a hypertensive effect (see Chapter 16).

Alcohol

Concomitant ingestion of alcohol with indoramin can increase the rate and extent of absorption of indoramin and increase its sedative effects.[6]

Antidepressants and antipsychotics

Antidepressants and antipsychotics may enhance the hypotensive effect of prazosin and other alpha blockers. Indoramin should not be given to patients who are already receiving monoamine oxidase inhibitors (MAOIs). Acute agitation developed in a patient taking chlorpromazine and amitriptyline when prazosin was added to therapy; symptoms settled rapidly on withdrawal of prazosin.

Antihypertensive drugs

Combination with other antihypertensives produces additive effects that are generally beneficial, although combination with a thiazide, beta blocker or calcium-channel blocker may increase the risk of first-dose hypotension and extra caution is required on initiating treatment. A markedly enhanced hypotensive effect has been reported in normotensive subjects given prazosin and verapamil concurrently, possibly due to enhanced bioavailability of prazosin.

Digoxin

Addition of prazosin therapy to patients receiving a maintenance dose of digoxin has been reported to increase the mean plasma digoxin concentration.

Preparations

See Table 11.1.

References

1. Nash D T. Alpha-adrenergic blockers: mechanism of action, blood pressure control, and effects on lipoprotein metabolism. *Clin Cardiol* 1990; 13: 764–772.
2. Young R A, Brogden R N. Doxazosin: a review of its pharmacodynamic and pharmacokinetic properties, and therapeutic efficacy in mild or moderate hypertension. *Drugs* 1988; 35: 524–541.
3. Carruthers S G. Adverse effects of α_1-adrenergic blocking drugs. *Drug Safety* 1994; 11: 12–20.
4. Marshall H J, Beevers D G. α-Adrenoceptor blocking drugs and female urinary incontinence: prevalence and reversibility. *Br J Clin Pharmacol* 1996; 42: 507–509.
5. Stockley I H. *Drug Interactions*, 5th edn. London: Pharmaceutical Press, 1999.
6. Abrams S M L, Pierce D M, Johnston A. Pharmacokinetic interaction between indoramin and ethanol. *Hum Toxicol* 1989; 8: 237–241.

12

Angiotensin II receptor antagonists

Indications

Angiotensin II receptor antagonists are a useful alternative for patients who have to discontinue an angiotensin-converting enzyme (ACE) inhibitor because of persistent cough. Beyond this, their role in hypertension remains to be established.

Mechanism of action[1,2]

Angiotensin II receptor antagonists, like ACE inhibitors (see Chapter 9), act on the renin–angiotensin system. Their development began in the early 1970s when the first peptide receptor antagonists of angiotensin II were described. However, being peptides, they had to be given by the intravenous route, which does not make them suitable for development as antihypertensive agents. It was not until a few years ago that the first of the orally active angiotensin II receptor antagonists, losartan (see Figure 12.1), reached the market. These orally active drugs are nonpeptide imidazole derivatives.

Angiotensin II receptor antagonists act as competitive antagonists of angiotensin II at angiotensin type 1 (AT_1) receptors. The major physiological effects of angiotensin II (the primary vasoactive hormone of the renin–angiotensin–aldosterone system) are vasoconstriction, stimulation of aldosterone secretion, regulation of salt and water homeostasis and stimulation of cell growth. These effects are mediated via the type 1 receptor that is found in many tissues (vascular smooth muscle, adrenal gland, kidneys and heart). Blockade of AT_1 receptors reduces the pressor effect of angiotensin II and reduces systemic peripheral resistance without a reflex increase in heart rate. Levels of the sodium-retaining hormone, aldosterone, are also reduced. Blockade of AT_1 receptors removes angiotensin II-negative feedback on renin secretion and therefore produces an increase in plasma renin levels. The increased plasma renin activity in turn produces an increase in angiotensin II plasma levels. However, despite these increases, the antihypertensive effect is maintained.

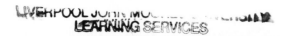

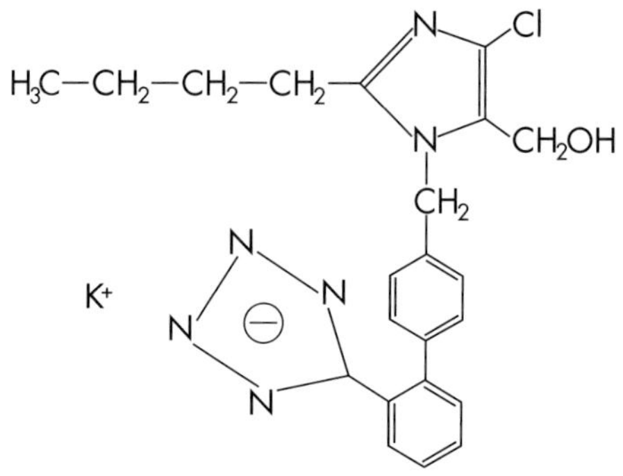

Figure 12.1 Losartan potassium.

As angiotensin II receptor antagonists do not inhibit the break-down of bradykinin and other kinins they do not appear to cause the persistent dry cough that commonly complicates ACE inhibitor therapy.[3] However, they may lack the additional physiological benefits that rises in bradykinin levels may bring, such as additional hypotensive effect. As with the ACE inhibitors, there is evidence that angiotensin II receptor antagonists may improve proteinuria.

All the angiotensin II receptor antagonists available (see Table 12.1) produce blood pressure lowering effects that last for at least 24 hours, so all are suitable for once-a-day administration. The maximal blood pressure lowering effect of a dose is usually seen within about 4–6 weeks.

Pharmacokinetics[4,5]

All of the angiotensin II receptor antagonists currently available are given orally. Candesartan cilexetil is an ester prodrug that is converted to the active moiety, candesartan, by ester hydrolysis during absorption from the gastrointestinal tract. Losartan has some activity as an angiotensin II receptor antagonist but undergoes hepatic metabolism to form an active carboxylic acid metabolite that has greater activity. The other angiotensin II receptor antagonists are administered as the active drug. All are highly bound to plasma proteins. All undergo some excretion in the bile; telmisartan and valsartan are excreted almost exclusively by this route (see Table 12.1).

Table 12.1 Angiotensin II receptor antagonists

Angiotensin II receptor antagonist	Half-life (h)	Elimination	Daily dose	Tablet strength (mg)	Comments	Proprietary name(s) (UK)	Manufacturer(s) (UK)
Candesartan cilexetil	9 (candesartan)	Hydrolysed to candesartan; excreted mainly unchanged in urine and bile	4 mg initially (2 mg in hepatic or renal impairment), adjusted according to response; usual maintenance dose 8 mg; max. 16 mg	2, 4, 8 and 16	A prodrug, rapidly converted to active drug candesartan by ester hydrolysis during absorption from the gastrointestinal tract. Contraindicated in severe hepatic impairment and cholestasis	Amias	Astra, Takeda
Eprosartan	5–9	Some metabolism; excreted in urine (mostly unchanged) and faeces	600 mg initially, increased if necessary after 2–3 weeks to 800 mg	300, 400 and 600 (as mesilate)	Reduce initial dose to 300 mg in elderly (>75 years), mild to moderate hepatic impairment or renal impairment. Contraindicated in severe hepatic impairment	Teveten	Solvay

continued overleaf

Table 12.1 Contd.

Angiotensin II receptor antagonist	Half-life (h)	Elimination	Daily dose	Tablet strength (mg)	Comments	Proprietary name(s) (UK)	Manufacturer(s) (UK)
Irbesartan	11–15	Metabolised in liver; excreted in bile (80%) and urine (20%)	150 mg, increased if necessary to 300 mg	75, 150 and 300	Reduce initial dose to 75 mg in patients on haemodialysis or in elderly (>75 years)	Aprovel	Bristol-Myers Squibb, Sanofi-Synthelabo
Losartan potassium	2 (losartan), 6–9 (carboxylic acid metabolite)	Extensively metabolised to carboxylic acid metabolite that has greater activity than losartan; excreted in bile (60%) and urine (35%)	50 mg initially, increased if necessary after several weeks to 100 mg	25 and 50	Reduce initial dose to 25 mg in elderly (>75 years), in moderate to severe renal impairment or in intravascular volume depletion	Cozaar	MSD

Table 12.1 Contd.

Angiotensin II receptor antagonist	Half-life (h)	Elimination	Daily dose	Tablet strength (mg)	Comments	Proprietary name(s) (UK)	Manufacturer(s) (UK)
Telmisartan	>20	Metabolised by glucuronide conjugation; excreted largely in bile	40 mg initially, increased if necessary to 80 mg	40 and 80	Contraindicated in biliary obstructive disorders and severe renal or hepatic impairment	Micardis	Boehringer-Ingelheim
Valsartan	5–9	No significant metabolism; excreted mainly in faeces	80 mg initially, increased if necessary after at least 4 weeks to 160 mg (80 mg in hepatic impairment)	40, 80 and 160	Reduce initial dose to 40 mg in elderly (>75 years), in mild to moderate hepatic impairment, in moderate to severe renal impairment or in intravascular volume depletion. Contraindicated in severe hepatic impairment or biliary obstruction	Diovan	Novartis

Dosage

See Table 12.1.

Adverse effects

Adverse effects have been reported to be usually mild and transient.[6] Like the ACE inhibitors (see Chapter 9), angiotensin II receptor antagonists may cause renal impairment and hypotension and special caution is necessary in certain patients (see Adverse Effects Focus, below). Hypotension may particularly occur in patients with salt or volume depletion and this should be corrected before treatment with angiotensin II receptor antagonists is started. Hypotension is minimised by starting treatment with a low dose. Also, like ACE inhibitors, angiotensin II receptor antagonists may cause hyperkalaemia; monitoring of serum potassium concentrations is recommended in the elderly and in patients with renal impairment or heart failure. The concomitant use of potassium-sparing diuretics or other agents that increase potassium concentrations should be avoided (see Drug interactions, below).

ADVERSE EFFECTS FOCUS

Cautions for the use of angiotensin II receptor antagonists

- Renal artery stenosis – increased risk of severe hypotension and renal insufficiency
- Impaired renal function – periodic monitoring of renal function and serum potassium concentrations is recommended. Some angiotensin II receptor antagonists are contraindicated in severe renal impairment (see Table 12.1)
- Salt/volume-depleted patients (those taking high-dose diuretics, those with vomiting or diarrhoea, salt-restricted patients) – increased risk of hypotension
- Elderly – increased risk of hypotension and hyperkalaemia (monitor serum potassium concentrations)
- Severe hepatic impairment – some angiotensin II receptor antagonists are contraindicated (see Table 12.1)
- Biliary obstruction or cholestasis – some angiotensin II receptor antagonists are contraindicated (see Table 12.1)
- Aortic stenosis or obstructive hypertrophic cardiomyopathy – a fall in blood pressure can aggravate these conditions

As mentioned under Mechanism of action, above, angiotensin II receptor antagonists do not increase bradykinin levels and therefore appear less likely than ACE inhibitors to cause cough. It was hoped that they would not be associated with angioedema, which is possibly caused by increased bradykinin levels; however, there are reports of angioedema occurring with some angiotensin II receptor antagonists.[7]

Other side-effects that have been reported include headache, fatigue, upper respiratory tract symptoms, muscle and joint pain, nausea, flushing, effects on the skin, anaemia, neutropenia and altered liver function tests. Telmisartan has caused gastrointestinal disturbances, including, rarely, gastrointestinal bleeding.

Drug interactions[8]

The antihypertensive effect of angiotensin II receptor antagonists is enhanced by concomitant administration with other drugs that have a secondary hypotensive effect and antagonised by administration with other drugs that have a hypertensive effect (see Chapter 16).

Hyperkalaemic effect enhanced

The risk of hyperkalaemia is increased if angiotensin II receptor antagonists are used in combination with other agents that increase potassium concentrations, such as potassium supplements, potassium-sparing diuretics, salt substitutes containing potassium or drugs that increase potassium concentrations such as indometacin and ciclosporin.

Lithium

As with ACE inhibitors (see p. 100), there is a possibility that concomitant use of an angiotensin II receptor antagonist with lithium could result in higher serum lithium concentrations.

Preparations

See Table 12.1.

References

1.   Goodfriend T L, Elliott M E, Catt K J. Angiotensin receptors and their antagonists. *N Engl J Med* 1996; 334: 1649–1654.

2. Burnier M, Brunner H R. Angiotensin II receptor antagonists. *Lancet* 2000; 355: 637–645.

3. Johnston C I. Angiotensin receptor antagonists: focus on losartan. *Lancet* 1995; 346: 1403–1407.

4. Csajka C, Buclin T, Brunner H R, Biollaz J. Pharmacokinetic–pharmacodynamic profile of angiotensin II receptor antagonists. *Clin Pharmacokinet* 1997; 32: 1–29.

5. Schaefer K L, Porter J A. Angiotensin II receptor antagonists: the prototype losartan. *Ann Pharmacother* 1996; 30: 625–636.

6. Mazzolai L, Burnier M. Comparative safety and tolerability of angiotensin II receptor antagonists. *Drug Safety* 1999; 21: 23–33.

7. Acker C G, Greenberg A. Angioedema induced by the angiotensin II blocker losartan. *N Engl J Med* 1995; 333: 1572.

8. Stockley I H. *Drug Interactions*, 5th edn. London: Pharmaceutical Press, 1999.

13

Miscellaneous antihypertensive drugs

In addition to the main groups of antihypertensive drugs, there are several other drugs that are useful for certain patients. Some of these are older drugs that were available before the major antihypertensives were discovered. While side-effects are a problem with some of these drugs, they may still be useful for some patients. Brief information on the action and major side-effects of these drugs is given below. Dosage information is given in Table 13.1. For more detailed information, see the *British National Formulary*[1] or *Martindale*.[2]

Loop diuretics

These include:

- Bumetanide
- Furosemide (frusemide)
- Torasemide.

Mechanism of action and indications

Loop diuretics are potent diuretics that act primarily on the ascending part of the loop of Henle and inhibit the reabsorption of electrolytes. They increase secretion of sodium, potassium, calcium and chloride ions. They have no clinically significant effect on carbonic anhydrase. They produce a brisk but short-lived diuresis. They have a role in patients with impaired renal function in whom thiazides may be ineffective, and in patients with hypertension resistant to multiple drug therapy, who are often fluid-overloaded.

Adverse effects

Fluid and electrolyte imbalance is the most common side-effect associated with loop diuretics. See Chapter 7 on thiazide diuretics for the symptoms and signs associated with electrolyte imbalance. Electrolyte

Table 13.1 Miscellaneous antihypertensive drugs

Drug group	Half-life (h)	Daily dose	Tablet strength (mg)	Comments	Proprietary name(s) (UK)	Manufacturer(s) (UK)
LOOP DIURETICS						
Bumetanide	1–2	0.5–2 mg	1 and 5	Oral liquid and injection also available. May cause muscle pain, particularly at high doses	Burinex	APS, Bioglan, Cox, CP, Genus, Hillcross, Leo, Norton
Furosemide (frusemide)	2	40–80 mg	20, 40 and 500	Oral liquid and injection also available	Froop, Lasix, Rusyde	APS, Ashbourne, Borg, Cox, CP, Hillcross, Norton, Sovereign
Torasemide	3.5	2.5 mg, increased if necessary to 5 mg	2.5, 5 and 10		Torem	Roche
POTASSIUM-SPARING DIURETICS						
Amiloride hydrochloride	20	5–10 mg initially	5	Oral liquid also available	Amilospare	APS, Ashbourne, Cox, CP, Hillcross, Norton Pharmark
Triamterene	2	50 mg initially (in combination with diuretic)	50	Give in divided doses after breakfast and lunch. May give urine a slight blue coloration	Dytac	
CENTRALLY ACTING ANTIHYPERTENSIVES						
Clonidine hydrochloride	6–24	150–300 µg (in three divided doses) increased every second or third day; usual max. 1.2 mg	100 and 300 µg	A modified-release preparation also available. Tolerance may occur. Withdrawal must be gradual	Catapres	Boehringer Ingelheim

Table 13.1 Contd.

Drug group	Half-life (h)	Daily dose	Tablet strength (mg)	Comments	Proprietary name(s) (UK)	Manufacturer(s) (UK)
Methyldopa		500–750 mg (given in two or three divided doses), gradually increased at intervals of 2 or more days; max. 3 g	125, 250 and 500	Elderly 125 mg twice daily initially, gradually increased; max. 2 g daily	Aldomet	Cox, CP, Hillcross, MSD, Norton, Sovereign
Moxonidine	2–3	200 µg, increased if necessary after 3 weeks to 400 µg (may be given in two divided doses); max. 600 µg (in two divided doses; max. single dose 400 µg)	200 and 400 µg	Give in the morning. Half-life prolonged in renal impairment; reduce dose	Physiotens	Solvay

continued overleaf

Table 13.1 Contd.

Drug group	Half-life (h)	Daily dose	Tablet strength (mg)	Comments	Proprietary name(s) (UK)	Manufacturer(s) (UK)
DIRECT VASODILATORS						
Hydralazine hydrochloride	2–4	50 mg increased to usual max. 100 mg	25	Daily dose given in two divided doses. Half-life prolonged in renal impairment	Apresoline	Alliance
Minoxidil	4	5 mg initially (elderly 2.5 mg), increased by 5–10 mg every 3 or more days; usual max. 50 mg	2.5, 5 and 10	Daily dose can be given as single dose or in two divided doses	Loniten	Pharmacia & Upjohn
ADRENERGIC NEURONE BLOCKERS						
Debrisoquine		10–20 mg, increased by 10 mg every 3 days; usual range 20–60 mg (120 mg or higher in severe hypertension)	10 (as sulphate)	Metabolism is subject to genetic polymorphism		Cambridge
Guanethidine monosulphate				Only the injection available in UK		

disturbances produced may include hyponatraemia, hypokalaemia and hypochloraemic alkalosis. These disturbances may occur particularly during chronic administration or with large doses. Loop diuretics may also cause hyperuricaemia and precipitate attacks of gout in some patients.

Other side-effects are relatively uncommon and include effects on the eyes, dizziness, headache, orthostatic hypotension, skin rashes, hypersensitivity reactions, bone marrow depression, pancreatitis, cholestatic jaundice, tinnitus and deafness.

Potassium-sparing diuretics

These include:

- Amiloride
- Triamterene.

Mechanism of action and indications

Potassium-sparing diuretics are weak diuretics acting mainly on the distal renal tubules to increase the excretion of sodium and reduce the excretion of potassium. They do not inhibit carbonic anhydrase. They have little effect on blood pressure. Potassium-sparing diuretics are mainly used as an adjunct to thiazide diuretics and loop diuretics to conserve potassium in those at risk from hypokalaemia (see p. 63). Potassium supplements must not be given with potassium-sparing diuretics. Administration of a potassium-sparing diuretic to a patient receiving an angiotensin-converting enzyme (ACE) inhibitor can also cause severe hyperkalaemia.

Spironolactone is another potassium-sparing diuretic that was formerly used, similarly to amiloride and triamterene, in hypertension. It acts on the distal portion of the renal tubule as a competitive antagonist of aldosterone. However, it is no longer used for patients with essential hypertension as there are doubts over its safety with long-term use.

Adverse effects

Potassium-sparing diuretics can cause hyperkalaemia. Elderly patients, diabetics and patients with impaired renal function are likely to be particularly affected. Hyponatraemia may also occur. Other side-effects include gastrointestinal disturbances, paraesthesia, thirst, dizziness, skin disorders, weakness, muscle cramps, headache and minor psychiatric or visual changes. Orthostatic hypotension and rises in blood urea nitrogen concentrations have been reported. Additional side-effects that may occur with triamterene include photosensitivity reactions, increases in uric acid concentrations, blood dyscrasias, renal calculi (in susceptible patients), megaloblastic anaemia (in patients with depleted folic acid stores) and reversible renal failure.

Centrally acting antihypertensives

These include:

* Clonidine
* Methyldopa
* Moxonidine.

Mechanism of action and indications

These drugs act centrally to reduce sympathetic tone, resulting in a fall in diastolic and systolic blood pressure and a reduction in heart rate. Peripheral resistance is reduced during continuous treatment. Stimulation of alpha$_2$-adrenoceptors is responsible for some of the effects. Clonidine also stimulates central imidazoline receptors. Methyldopa is decarboxylated in the central nervous system to alpha-methylnoradrenaline, thought to stimulate alpha$_2$-adrenoceptors. Methyldopa may also act as a false neurotransmitter and reduce plasma renin activity. Moxonidine is a new centrally acting drug that has recently been introduced. It is structurally related to clonidine and acts on central imidazoline receptors to reduce sympathetic tone. It also has some alpha$_2$-adrenoceptor agonist activity.

Clonidine was extensively used in the past to treat hypertension but has largely been superseded by the newer classes of antihypertensives that have fewer side-effects. Clonidine is also used intravenously in hypertensive crises. Methyldopa is commonly used in hypertensive pregnant women. Moxonidine may have a role when the main antihypertensive drugs are contraindicated or not tolerated or fail to control blood pressure.

Reserpine and rauwolfia are also centrally acting antihypertensive drugs. They are no longer used in the UK.

Adverse effects

Clonidine and methyldopa cause drowsiness, dry mouth, dizziness and headache, especially during the initial stages of therapy; fluid retention may also occur. Clonidine also commonly causes constipation and has the disadvantage that sudden withdrawal may cause a hypertensive crisis. This rebound hypertension may be exacerbated by beta blockers and, if a beta blocker is given concurrently with clonidine, clonidine should not be discontinued until several days after the withdrawal of the beta blocker.

Methyldopa can also cause hypersensitivity reactions, including haemolytic anaemia and disturbances of liver function.

Moxonidine has similar adverse effects to clonidine but causes less sedation and possibly less dry mouth.

Direct vasodilators

These include:

- Hydralazine
- Minoxidil.

Mechanism of action and indications

These agents act directly to relax vascular smooth muscle, thereby reducing peripheral vascular resistance. They act predominantly on the arterioles. The reduction in peripheral resistance produces a reflex tachycardia and increased cardiac output. Hydralazine also tends to improve renal and cerebral blood flow and its effect on diastolic pressure is more marked than on systolic pressure.

Hydralazine and minoxidil are given orally in hypertension in combination with other agents (a beta blocker or methyldopa and a diuretic) to reduce the tachycardia and fluid retention that occur when they are used alone. Minoxidil is reserved for severe hypertension unresponsive to standard therapy. Hydralazine is also given intravenously in hypertensive crises.

Diazoxide and sodium nitroprusside are other direct vasodilators. Diazoxide is restricted to administration by intravenous injection in hypertensive emergencies. It is not suitable for chronic treatment of hypertension because of the severity of the adverse effects it produces. Sodium nitroprusside is given by intravenous infusion to control severe hypertensive crises on the rare occasions when parenteral treatment is necessary.

Adverse effects

As mentioned above, both hydralazine and minoxidil cause tachycardia and fluid retention. Other side-effects occurring frequently with hydralazine include angina pectoris, severe headache and gastro-intestinal disturbances (anorexia, nausea, vomiting and diarrhoea). These side-effects are seen particularly at the start of treatment, and especially if the dose is increased quickly. They generally subside with continued treatment. With prolonged treatment and high doses, a condition resembling systemic lupus erythematosus may develop and should be suspected if there is unexplained weight loss, arthritis or any other unexplained ill health. The incidence is greater in patients taking more than 100 mg of hydralazine daily.

Other common side-effects of minoxidil include oedema and sometimes deterioration of existing heart failure and changes in the electro-cardiogram. Hypertrichosis develops in up to 80% of patients within 3–6 weeks of starting treatment, which makes it an unsuitable drug for use in women. The hypertrichosis is slowly reversible on discontinuation of treatment.

Adrenergic neurone blockers

These include:

- Debrisoquine
- Guanethidine.

Mechanism of action and indications

Adrenergic neurone blocking drugs prevent the release of noradrenaline (norepinephrine) from postganglionic adrenergic neurones. Guanethidine also causes the depletion of noradrenaline stores in peripheral sympathetic nerve terminals. Debrisoquine causes less depletion of noradrenaline stores. They produce an initial reduction in cardiac output but their main hypotensive effect is to cause peripheral vasodilatation. In the majority of patients they reduce standing blood pressure but have a less marked effect on supine blood pressure. These drugs may cause postural hypotension and for this reason they have fallen largely from use. They may be used, mainly in conjunction with other antihypertensives, in resistant hypertension. Guanethidine may be given parenterally in the management of hypertensive crises.

Adverse effects

The most common side-effects are severe postural hypotension and exertional hypotension. Hypotension may be particularly troublesome during the initial stages of therapy and during dose adjustment. It may be severe enough to cause angina, signs of renal insufficiency and transient cerebral ischaemia. Diarrhoea is also common with guanethidine during the initial stages of treatment. Other frequent side-effects are bradycardia, failure of ejaculation, fatigue, headache, salt and water retention and oedema.

Abrupt withdrawal of debrisoquine must be avoided as rebound hypertension can occur.

Preparations

See Table 13.1.

References

1. Mehta D K, ed. *British National Formulary*, no. 40. London: British Medical Association/RPSGB, 2000.
2. Parfitt K, ed. *Martindale: The Complete Drug Reference*, 32nd edn. London: Pharmaceutical Press, 1999.

14

New therapies and future developments

Current areas of research in hypertension include: the development of novel antihypertensive agents; identification of genetic factors in essential hypertension; blood pressure targets for different high-risk groups; and combined interventions to prevent cardiovascular disease.

Novel antihypertensive drugs

Some of the antihypertensive agents under investigation include endothelin receptor antagonists, renin inhibitors and potassium-channel openers.

Endothelin receptor antagonists

Endothelin$_1$ is a very potent vasoconstrictor peptide that was discovered in 1988. It is produced in a wide variety of tissues, including the vascular endothelium. Some studies have found that patients with essential hypertension have elevated plasma levels of endothelin$_1$, although other studies have found no elevation. Several endothelin receptors have been identified and various endothelin receptor antagonists are under development. One non-peptide compound, bosentan, that is given orally, is an antagonist at endothelin$_A$ and endothelin$_B$ receptors. A study in patients with essential hypertension found that it produced significant blood pressure lowering.[1]

Renin inhibitors

Renin catalyses the conversion of angiotensinogen to angiotensin I, the precursor of the vasoconstrictor angiotensin II. Inhibition of renin would therefore be expected to have a blood pressure lowering effect. Renin inhibitors would have the advantage of inhibiting production of angiotensin I and II without increasing the renin release that occurs following use of angiotensin-converting enzyme (ACE) inhibitors or angiotensin II receptor antagonists. A problem in the development of renin inhibitors has been developing an orally active drug. Enalkiren has been shown to have an antihypertensive effect in patients with hypertension, but it is a dipeptide that has to be given intravenously. This makes it an unlikely candidate for use in hypertension management. Other orally active renin inhibitors, such as remikiren, are under development.[2]

Potassium-channel openers

Potassium-channel openers (also known as potassium-channel activators) have a direct relaxant effect on smooth muscle, producing vasodilatation in blood vessels. The relaxation of smooth muscle occurs when the potassium-channel activator causes the efflux of potassium from smooth muscle cells, thus producing hyperpolarisation of the cell membrane. This leads to a reduction in intracellular calcium that in turn produces smooth muscle relaxation. Pinacidil is an orally active potassium-channel opener under investigation in hypertension.[3] The peripheral vasodilatation it produces provokes a reflex tachycardia and increase in cardiac output. It also causes fluid retention. Other potassium-channel openers under investigation include cromakalim and its (–)-enantiomer levcromakalim.

Genetic factors

Genetic analysis is being used to try and unravel the genetic basis of essential hypertension. It is thought that by the time most cases of essential hypertension are diagnosed, much of the structural damage in the heart and blood vessels that is responsible for the complications of hypertension has already occurred. Many cases of essential hypertension will be due to interactions between genetic and environmental factors. However, it is hoped that more monogenic syndromes can be identified and that this will allow selection of optimal treatment and accurate prediction of prognosis. Identification of these syndromes could also lead to the development of novel antihypertensive agents and may allow intervention before the irreversible structural changes have occurred.[4]

Blood pressure targets

Results from the UKPDS study[5] and the HOT study[6] provide evidence that diabetic patients with hypertension gain important reductions in cardiovascular risk by reducing blood pressure to a lower target pressure.

It is hoped that further research can identify whether other high-risk groups with hypertension would benefit similarly from lower blood pressure targets.

Combined interventions to prevent cardiovascular disease

The recognition that blood pressure reduction must occur in the context of control of overall cardiovascular risk has led to more emphasis on combined treatment with antiplatelets and statins in addition to antihypertensive drugs. Further research is needed to clarify which patients stand to benefit from these treatments and whether other agents may be of use in reducing cardiovascular risk, such as folic acid for lowering homocysteine levels.

References

1. Krum H, Viskoper R J, Lacourciere Y, *et al*. The effect of an endothelin-receptor antagonist, bosentan, on blood pressure in patients with essential hypertension. *N Engl J Med* 1998; 338: 784–790.
2. Frishman W H, Fozailoff A, Lin C, Dike C. Renin inhibition: a new approach to cardiovascular therapy. *J Clin Pharmacol* 1994; 34: 873–880.
3. Friedel H A, Brogden R N. Pinacidil: a review of its pharmacodynamic and pharmacokinetic properties, and therapeutic potential in the treatment of hypertension. *Drugs* 1990; 39: 929–967.
4. Brown M J. Hypertension. *BMJ* 1997; 314: 1258–1261.
5. UK Prospective Diabetes Study Group. Tight blood pressure control and risk of macrovascular and microvascular complications in type 2 diabetes: UKPDS 38. *BMJ* 1998; 317: 703–713. Correction *ibid*. 1999; 318: 29.
6. Hansson L, Zanchetti A, Carruthers S G, *et al*. Effects of intensive blood-pressure lowering and low-dose aspirin in patients with hypertension: principal results of the Hypertension Optimal Treatment (HOT) randomised trial. *Lancet* 1998; 351: 1755–1762.

15

Primary prevention and screening

Primary prevention[1]

Primary prevention forms an important part of the management of hypertension, since there are several aspects of current treatment that are unsatisfactory.

- A significant proportion of cardiovascular disease occurs in people whose blood pressure is higher than the optimal level (120/80 mmHg) but lower than that diagnosed as hypertensive (140/90 mmHg).
- The current management strategy for hypertension involves the detection and lifelong drug therapy of a large proportion of the adult population with the associated financial costs and adverse effects.
- Many patients do not comply with drug therapy or make the necessary life-style changes.
- Despite treatment, hypertensives still have a higher cardiovascular risk than normotensive people do.

The aims of primary prevention strategies are summarised in Management Focus, below.

There is increasing evidence that a population strategy could prevent the rise in blood pressure with age, reduce the prevalence of hypertension and need for drug therapy, and reduce overall cardiovascular risk. Primary prevention aims to shift the whole blood pressure distribution to the left by altering the general population lifestyle. Only

MANAGEMENT FOCUS

Aims of primary prevention

- Lower the blood pressure by a few degrees in the entire population and therefore reduce the number of cardiovascular events
- Prevent the age-related rise in blood pressure
- Increase awareness of hypertension and thereby increase screening
- Reduce the need for drugs in patients with hypertension

a small reduction in blood pressure is required to produce a surprisingly large decrease in cardiovascular risk. It has been estimated that a 2 mmHg downward shift in the entire distribution of systolic blood pressure is likely to reduce the annual mortality from stroke by 6%, coronary heart disease by 4% and all causes by 3%.

A population approach is based on lifestyle modifications that have been shown to prevent or delay blood pressure rise in susceptible people. These lifestyle changes are described in Chapter 6. Pharmacists have an important part to play in primary prevention since they are ideally placed to provide information on lifestyle issues such as diet, exercise, alcohol consumption and stress. The provision of smoking cessation advice and cholesterol screening services is also important.

Better public understanding about hypertension, its causes and consequences forms an important part of primary prevention. Such information can help people understand the importance of making changes to their lifestyles. However, attempting to change people's behaviour requires a sustained education campaign that targets all sections of the community and all ages and that is consistently promoted by health care professionals and the media. Since primary prevention provides only a relatively small preventive benefit to each individual, particularly in the short term, generating sufficient motivation for people to make lifestyle changes can be difficult. Therefore it is important that modifications that do not rely on people's compliance, such as reducing salt content of processed foods, are also pursued.

Screening for hypertension

There are no reliable signs or symptoms that indicate the presence of hypertension; headache may sometimes be a symptom but generally only when diastolic blood pressure is very severely elevated (>130 mmHg). Thus, screening is an essential part of hypertension management so that those with elevated blood pressure can receive treatment before a cardiovascular event intervenes. Although mass screening is not feasible, every opportunity should be taken to measure blood pressure during regular health care encounters. The British Hypertension Society (BHS) recommends[2] that all adults should have their blood pressure measured every 5 years and that this should continue up until the age of 80 years. If a high-normal reading is found at any time (135–139/85–89 mmHg) then more frequent re-measurements should be made (the BHS recommends annually[2]). Doctors should explain to patients the meaning of their blood pressure readings and advise them of the need for periodic re-measurement. Increasing public awareness of hypertension should encourage self-referral.

Community pharmacists can help by providing blood pressure measuring facilities for screening. They may also be involved in monitoring blood pressure as part of the management of patients with hypertension. The Pharmaceutical Society's guidelines[3] give useful information on setting up a service in community pharmacy. The importance of accurate blood pressure measurement and the procedure that should be followed are discussed in Chapter 3.

References

1. WHO. Hypertension control: report of a WHO Expert Committee. *WHO Tech Rep Ser 862.* 1996.
2. Ramsay L E, Williams B, Johnston G D, *et al.* BHS guidelines. Guidelines for management of hypertension: report of the third working party of the British Hypertension Society. *J Hum Hypertens* 1999; 13: 569–592.
3. Snell M, ed. *Medicines, Ethics and Practice 24: A Guide for Pharmacists.* London: RPSGB, July 2000.

16

Pharmaceutical assessment of the hypertensive patient

As discussed in the introduction (Chapter 1), many patients diagnosed as having hypertension fail to gain the benefits they should from their treatment and go on to develop complications of hypertension. Many factors contribute to this treatment failure; compliance problems, poor patient education and inadequate follow-up are central features. These are all areas where intervention by a pharmacist can make a significant difference. Patients with hypertension often have more regular contact with the pharmacist than any other health care professional. By putting into practice the principles of medicines management (or pharmaceutical care), pharmacists can be expected to help patients with hypertension achieve improved clinical outcomes.[1]

Some of the issues the pharmacist will need to consider are listed in the Management Focus (see p. 152).

Cholesterol measurement

Blood cholesterol concentration, along with elevated blood pressure and smoking, is one of the most important risk factors for cardiovascular disease. Blood cholesterol measurement may be offered in the pharmacy as a screening service but it may also be useful for those patients assigned to a lipid-lowering therapy or diet as a means of assessing compliance with treatment. It may also form part of a patient's ongoing assessment of overall cardiovascular risk. The Royal Pharmaceutical Society's Code of ethics[2] includes guidelines on the setting-up of such a service.

General dietary recommendations for a healthy diet include reducing fat intake (total fat intake should not exceed 30% of total daily calories), substituting monounsaturated or polyunsaturated fats for saturated fats and increasing consumption of fibre (vegetables, fruit, cereals and bread). The importance of exercise, losing excess body weight and reducing excessive alcohol intake should also be stressed. Patients requiring a specific lipid-lowering diet should receive this advice from a dietician.

MANAGEMENT FOCUS

Medicines management in the hypertensive patient

- Education about hypertension and its consequences (Chapter 2)
- Contribution of risk factors and any existing cardiovascular disease (Chapter 3)
- Comorbidity affecting treatment (Chapters 4 and 5)
- Selection of appropriate drug (Chapters 4 and 5)
- Education about the drugs prescribed, including adverse effects (see relevant drug chapter)
- Tailoring drug regimen to suit patient's lifestyle
- Aims of treatment (Chapter 4)
- Blood pressure monitoring by pharmacist (Chapter 15)
- Advice on lifestyle measures (Chapter 6)
- Screening for cholesterol levels (see p. 151)
- Monitoring for adverse effects
- Looking out for drug interactions with prescribed medication and over-the-counter products (see below)
- Assessing compliance problems with drug therapy and lifestyle measures (see p. 154)
- Indications that stepdown of treatment may be needed

Interactions

Significant interactions specific to individual antihypertensive drug classes are covered under the relevant drug chapter.

Many drugs possess hypotensive or hypertensive effects. Risk Factor Focus (see p. 9) lists some of the drugs that can produce hypertension and that can counteract the effect of antihypertensive drugs. Some of the drugs that can produce hypotension are listed in the Risk Factor Focus (see p. 153). In some cases, combination of one of these agents with an antihypertensive drug may be beneficial, but caution is needed when the combination is introduced to avoid excessive hypotension.

NSAIDs

Non-steroidal anti-inflammatory drugs (NSAIDs) are very widely used agents and may be prescribed for a patient with hypertension or they may be requested over-the-counter (OTC). NSAIDs can raise blood pressure, generally by only a few mmHg,[3] although there is considerable individual variability and the increase could be significant in some

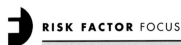

Drugs that can produce hypotension
Alcohol
Aldesleukin
Alprostadil
Anaesthetics, general
Antiarrhythmics (bretylium, procainamide, quinidine, tocainide)
Antidepressants (particularly monoamine oxidase inhibitors and tricyclics)
Antipsychotics
Anxiolytics
Contrast agents
Dopaminergics
Muscle relaxants
Nabilone (high-dose)
Nitrates
Opioid analgesics
Pentoxifylline
Phenothiazines

patients. The effects of most antihypertensive drugs are attenuated by concomitant administration with NSAIDs, with the possible exception of calcium-channel blockers.

Ibuprofen, indometacin, naproxen and piroxicam seem to produce the largest effect on blood pressure and aspirin, flurbiprofen and sulindac the smallest effect, although comparative data are scarce.[3,4] The mechanism of the interaction is probably inhibition of the synthesis of vasodilator prostaglandins, although sodium retention is also a factor. For more specific interactions between NSAIDs and angiotensin-converting enzyme (ACE) inhibitors, see Chapter 9.

OTC products

Some groups of OTC drugs have the potential to cause problems in patients with hypertension, either because of their effect on blood pressure or because of an interaction with an antihypertensive drug (see Adverse Effects Focus, p. 154).

Compliance

Non-compliance with both drug therapy and lifestyle measures is a major problem in hypertension management and pharmacists need to be

ADVERSE EFFECTS FOCUS

Potential problems with OTC medicines in hypertension

- Antacids: some antacids contain large amounts of sodium. These antacids may cause fluid retention and oppose the action of antihypertensive drugs. Patients with hypertension requiring an antacid should use the 'low-sodium' antacids available (<1 mmol sodium/dose)
   Antacids can reduce absorption of captopril, fosinopril and possibly other ACE inhibitors; their administration must be separated
- H$_2$-receptor antagonists: cimetidine may inhibit the metabolism of some calcium-channel blockers. An alternative H$_2$-receptor antagonist should be used
- Herbal preparations containing liquorice can cause fluid retention and counteract the action of antihypertensive drugs. Other herbal ingredients that can cause hypertension are listed in Risk Factor Focus (p. 9)
- Oral decongestants containing sympathomimetics such as ephedrine, pseudoephedrine and phenylpropanolamine should be used with caution in patients with hypertension as they may cause an increase in blood pressure due to release of noradrenaline (norepinephrine) from nerve endings. The combination of a nonselective beta blocker and oral decongestant could lead to a severe hypertensive reaction
- Topical decongestants (oxymetazoline, phenylephrine and xylometazoline) act mainly by a direct action on the blood vessels in the nose and are thus less likely than oral decongestants to affect blood pressure if used correctly. Patients should be counselled on how to use nose drops/sprays correctly so that they do not swallow any of the drug
- NSAIDs (see p. 152)
- Potassium-containing preparations. Salt substitutes may be requested by hypertensive patients who are advised to reduce their salt intake. They may produce hyperkalaemia in patients taking potassium-sparing diuretics or ACE inhibitors.
   Potassium citrate, used to treat dysuria, could cause hyperkalaemia in patients on potassium-sparing diuretics or ACE inhibitors

---

alert for signs of it. It is estimated that poor compliance contributes to lack of adequate control in more than two-thirds of patients. There are many factors that can contribute to non-compliance in hypertension, and some of these are listed in Management Focus, (see p. 155).

Some patients may be particularly prone to problems with compliance; elderly patients who are often taking many different medicines

MANAGEMENT FOCUS

Factors influencing compliance

- Lack of patient understanding about hypertension and need for treatment to prevent future complications
- Hypertension is usually asymptomatic and therefore the patient has little motivation to follow treatment
- Multiple daily doses
- Multiple drugs
- Side-effects
- Treatment must usually be continued for life
- Diagnosis can have job implications
- Many modifications to lifestyle may be needed to adhere to the recommended measures
- Lack of early subjective benefit of treatment

and are more likely to suffer confusion are particularly prone to poor compliance, as are others on multiple drugs or multiple daily doses. Good compliance is encouraged by keeping drug regimens as simple as possible, using long-acting once-daily preparations and combination preparations where appropriate. Patient education about the risks of hypertension and the need for long-term treatment and lifestyle measures is also important in providing a motivating factor for complying with treatment. Other motivating factors include having a clear goal of therapy and involving the patient by monitoring blood pressure at home. Pharmacists may also be involved in monitoring a patient's blood pressure and this provides an opportunity to reinforce the importance of compliance with drug and lifestyle measures. The effect of treatment on quality of life can be a major factor in compliance; pharmacists should be alert for side-effects, as many patients may accept them as part of the treatment and not realise other options are available. If adverse effects are a factor in poor compliance, then changing to another drug class should be attempted.

Compliance is a particular problem with lifestyle measures, especially as patients usually feel well to start with. Patients may need to make significant changes in their lifestyle and good advice and counselling are needed if they are to make the necessary changes. Enlisting family support is especially important in helping institute lifestyle changes and also helps with compliance with drug therapy.

References

1. Hudson S, McAnaw J, McGlynn S, Boyter A. Essential hypertension. *Pharm J* 1998; 260: 411–417.
2. Snell M, ed. *Medicines, Ethics and Practice 24: A Guide for Pharmacists.* London: RPSGB, 2000.
3. Johnson A G, Nguyen T V, Day R O. Do nonsteroidal anti-inflammatory drugs affect blood pressure? *Ann Intern Med* 1994; 121: 289–300.
4. Pope J E, Anderson J J, Felson D T. A meta-analysis of the effects of non-steroidal anti-inflammatory drugs on blood pressure. *Arch Intern Med* 1993; 153: 477–484.

Recommended reading

Textbooks and general references

Birkenhäger W H, ed. *Practical Management of Hypertension*, 2nd edn. Dordrecht: Kluwer Academic, 1996.

Centre for Pharmacy Postgraduate Education. *Hypertension; A Distance Learning Pack for Community Pharmacists*. Manchester: CPPE, 1993.

Centre for Pharmacy Postgraduate Education. *Hypertension and Hyperlipidaemia*. Manchester: CPPE, 1998.

Centre for Pharmacy Postgraduate Education. *Prescribing in Cardiovascular Diseases*. Manchester: CPPE, 1998.

Cipolle R J, Strand L M, Morley P C. *Pharmaceutical Care Practice*. New York: McGraw Hill, 1998.

Continuing Pharmacy Education. *New Drugs in Context: Hypertension Update*. Curtin: Pharmaceutical Society of Australia, 1999.

Kaplan N M. *Clinical Hypertension*, 7th edn. Baltimore, MD: Williams & Wilkins, 1998.

Mallarkey G, ed. *Aspects of Hypertension Management*. New Zealand: Adis International, 1999.

O'Brien E, Beevers D G, Marshall H J. *ABC of Hypertension*, 3rd edn. London: BMJ Publishing Group, 1995.

Opie L H, Messerli F H, eds. *Combination Drug Therapy for Hypertension*. New York: Lippincott-Raven, 1997.

Postel-Vinay N, ed. *A Century of Arterial Hypertension 1896–1996*. Chichester: John Wiley/Imothep, 1996.

Spencer C, Lip G. Hypertension. 1. Epidemiology and risks. *Pharm J* 1999; 263: 280–283.

Spencer C, Lip G. Hypertension. 2. Antihypertensive drugs. *Pharm J* 1999; 263: 351–354.

Spencer C, Lip G. Hypertension. 3. Management of the hypertensive patient. *Pharm J* 1999; 263: 383–386.

Spencer C, Lip G. Hypertension. 4. Recent advances in hypertension. *Pharm J* 1999; 263: 486–488.

Swales J D, ed. *Manual of Hypertension*. Oxford: Blackwell Science, 1995.

Hypertension in children

Bartosh S M, Aronson A J. Childhood hypertension: an update on etiology, diagnosis, and treatment. *Pediatr Clin North Am* 1999; 46: 235–252.

Deal J E, Barratt T M, Dillon M J. Management of hypertensive emergencies. *Arch Dis Child* 1992; 67: 1089–1092.

Hypertensive emergencies

Hirschl M M. Guidelines for the drug treatment of hypertensive crises. *Drugs* 1995; 50: 991–1000.

Kaplan N M. Management of hypertensive emergencies. *Lancet* 1994; 344: 1335–1338.

Hypertension in pregnancy

Broughton Pipkin F. The hypertensive disorders of pregnancy. *BMJ* 1995; 11: 609–613.

Brown M A, Whitworth J A. Management of hypertension in pregnancy. *Clin Exp Hypertens* 1999; 21: 907–916.

Gallery E D. Hypertension in pregnancy: practical management recommendations. *Drugs* 1995; 49: 555–562.

Kyle P M, Redman C W. Comparative risk–benefit assessment of drugs used in the management of hypertension in pregnancy. *Drug Safety* 1992; 7: 223–234.

Sibai B M. Treatment of hypertension in pregnant women. *N Engl J Med* 1996; 335: 257–265.

Teoh T G, Redman C W. Management of pre-existing disorders in pregnancy: hypertension. *Prescribers' J* 1996; 36: 28–36.

Hypertension in renal disease

Brown M A, Whitworth J A. Hypertension in human renal disease. *J Hypertens* 1992; 10: 701–712.

Derkx F H M, Schalekamp M A D H. Renal artery stenosis and hypertension. *Lancet* 1994; 344: 237–239.

Rosenthal T. Drug therapy of renovascular hypertension. *Drugs* 1993; 45: 895–909.

Index

Brand names are in *italic* type. Page numbers in **bold** refer to main discussions. Page numbers in *italics* refer to focus boxes, figures and tables.